TABLE OF

ACKNOWLEDGMENTS		2
Ch 1:	Experts	4
Ch 2:	Introducing the Medicine Man	17
Ch 3:	Who Told You That and Why Do You Believe Them	30
Ch 4:	Weeding Out the Garden	43
Ch 5:	Did Curiosity Kill the Cat or Make Him King of the Forest	61
Ch 6:	A Diploma Does Not a Doctor Make	74
Ch 7:	The Seed vs the Soil	82
Ch 8:	You Are What You Eat	100
Ch 9:	Milk, Calcium, Osteoporosis, and Allergies	112
Ch 10:	Choices	122
Ch 11:	Life vs Death. Not All Supplements Are Created Equal	134
Ch 12:	Synthetic Vitamins Are Not Vitamins at All	147
Ch 13:	Add Some Punch to Your Lunch	153
Ch 14:	Drink Up!	162
Ch 15:	Breath of Life	170
Ch 16:	Do You Mind if I Breathe While You Smoke?	178
Ch 17:	Couch Potatoes and Idiot Boxes	180
Ch 18:	Chiropractic: The Best Kept Secret on Earth	186
Ch 19:	Vaccines: A Toxic Shot Syndrome	199
Ch 20:	Acupuncture: New Age Medicine is Age Old Wisdom	226
Ch 21:	Look Out For the Boogeyman	239

ACKNOWLEDGMENTS

"There is one thing stronger than all the armies in the world and that is an idea whose time has come."
Victor Hugo

This book is a culmination of a lifetime of learning. Whether the learning has come through books, schools, personal research, seminars, life experience, group discussions, divine inspiration, or even a road trip with a friend, they have all enhanced my own understanding of life and death and what goes on in between. Through their actions and their wisdom, the following list of people has helped to create my paradigm of health and are, in part, responsible for the writing of this book. Though this list could in itself be as long as the book, I will mention only those who have had a profound influence on my perception of life and my role in it. These people have expanded my mind to such a degree that I can never again look at the world as I once did. They have taught me that every story has two sides to it even though politics, money, and special interests want you to believe otherwise. They have shown me a world filled with spirituality and wonder. These people have taught me to question everything until I find an answer that resonates with my soul, for it is here where the truth resides. They have helped me tap into a realm of existence that few people dream about and even fewer actually experience. For that, I am eternally grateful and say thank you to these paradigm-shifting mentors:

Weston Price, Deepak Chopra, Caroline Myss, Walene James, Robert Mendelsohn, Richard Gerber, Tom Brown, Ken Wilbur, Ken Pelletier, Peter Duesberg, and Marlo Morgan. Thanks also for the thoughts and lives of Albert Einstein, Joseph Campbell, Maxine McMullin, B.J. Palmer, Fred Barge, Edgar Cayce, Savannah Rae Kirsenlohr and Louis the Spotted Man,

Bruce Lipton, Royal Lee, and especially my family because they allow me the freedom to be myself.

I must also acknowledge our founding fathers who granted us the freedoms of speech and press in the first amendment to The Constitution of the United States. With our Bill of Rights, I am awarded the right to speak my mind freely and express my opinions. Without it, the information in this book might never have been allowed into print. I will undoubtedly upset some people, groups, and industries that do not understand life the way I do. My views are not conventional. My understanding of life is not steeped in profit. It is founded in service and gratitude. It is grounded in common sense and an enduring appreciation for the mystery that creates life.

This book is an interpretation of the information, education, facts, and life experiences I have been exposed to. Do the facts in this book explaining my interpretations of life and health make this information gospel? Of course it doesn't. They make this book my interpretation, my opinion, and nothing more. I ask you to apply an unbiased mind to these pages and see how the information fits your own paradigm. If my ideas rub you the wrong way, then continue living as you do now. If some of my points stimulate you to question the status quo and your role on this planet then embrace this book and see where it takes you. Thank you.

CHAPTER ONE

EXPERTS

"The problems that exist in the world today cannot be solved by the level of thinking that created them."
Albert Einstein

When it pertains to health care, there is a whirlwind of information constantly swirling around us and it is becoming more difficult to see through the chaos. Not a day goes by without one of my patients asking me what I know about a certain supplement, a particular diet, or the latest infomercial espousing the benefits of some cockamamie way to achieve optimal health. These people are confused and they are looking for answers. I cannot blame them. We have all, for as far back as we can remember, been assaulted by suggestions from the medical profession, celebrities, pharmaceutical companies, athletes, and assorted hucksters from every corner of the earth, through all forms of media, all telling us that Centrum is complete from A to Zinc, Zocor isn't right for everyone, and a simple contour pillow will restore our body's natural alignment. Is Larry King a consumer of Garlique or just a spokesman? What does Rush Limbaugh honestly know about Citracal? Does he have any education in nutrition or is he plugging for a sponsor? How did your brother loose 80 pounds using the Gazelle Elite but all you got was a backache? Does Joe Namath really find relief in using Flexall?

There are people who have tried electrocuting their abdominal muscles to develop a physique fit for the beach. Some say it worked. Some say it did not. An acquaintance had good success with chiropractic but your medical doctor says chiropractors are quacks. For eons of time, the herb Kava Kava has been used successfully to help reduce stress and anxiety. Not too long ago it was implicated by the medical establishment as causing liver dysfunction. Who can we believe? Did we receive all the data surrounding this news story or was much of it suppressed to create a bias? For instance, we were not told that this research was conducted with the wrong part of the Kava plant or that acetone was used as a solvent. Did the news piece include information as to how many of the reactions resulted from using Kava Kava in combination with pharmaceuticals? Some statements were factual but some statements were filled with fear-induced propaganda. With all this conflicting information, how can you trust the experts?

One young lady I spoke to was confined to a wheelchair. I was in a mall at the time and I approached her wishing to impart the powers of alternative medicine to her. I introduced myself and asked about her condition and what she was currently doing about it. As I started to communicate the wonders of acupuncture to her, she pulled back with a look in her eyes that was not at all friendly. She told me that the acupuncture needles are all made in China, and before they are shipped to the United States they are blessed by Satan. According to her sources, acupuncture is the work of the devil and I should abandon it altogether to save myself. This is an extreme example of misinformation but that kind of propaganda does exist in abundance today.

Copper bracelets, magnets, chelation, yoga, vaccines, grape-seed extract, colonics, Rolfing, creams to enhance breast size, shampoos to re-grow hair, Pilates, Noni Juice, Metabolife, Botox, colloidal minerals, antibiotics, Sea Silver, and DHEA supplements are just a few of the entities that are claimed to enhance our health in some fashion. The list goes on and on and on. Some claims hold merit. Some claims fail to live up to the hype. Some therapies are safe. With some therapies the benefits may not outweigh the risks. Some therapies are backed by scientific analysis but does scientific analysis really matter? Does science know everything there is to know about health? Are there some things science hasn't "proven" yet that are beneficial to us anyway?

Turning to so-called experts for answers will not provide much relief from the mayhem. Cutting-edge studies from prestigious research institutions can sound impressive but grandma's folk remedy for removing warts may in fact hold more merit. Not that long ago we were told that fat in butter was not good for us. It clogged arteries and lead to arteriosclerosis. Excess butter had a deleterious effect on cholesterol levels. The excess fat could lead to weight problems. Margarine became the savior but like all good saviors, it too, was soon sacrificed. We have since learned that the hydrogenated fats in margarine can damage the liver and cause more problems than butter. Margarine can lead to coronary heart disease, can decrease the immune response, and can create degenerative cellular changes. As if margarine wasn't bad enough, the powers that be unloaded Olestra, the fat substitute, onto our grocery store shelves. Olestra produced the same fat flavor without the added pounds. Olestra will, however, rob your body's supply of vitamins A, D, E, and K, cause gastrointestinal discomfort, excess gas, and anal leakage. Who is making these decisions and who is giving them justification?

Sugar has not evaded the firing squad either. For a while, sugar was the guilty party involved in weight management problems, diabetes, dental caries, and nervous tension. To combat this, the food-processing industry quickly invented the synthetic sweeteners Sweet and Low, Equal, and NutraSweet. Soon, Americans began adding those to shopping carts. Once again we were presented with contradiction. The Aspartame and saccharine in the artificial sweeteners have been implicated in altered brain chemistry, headaches, convulsions, and tumors. The Food and

Drug Administration has received more complaints about the side effects of aspartame than any other food additive in history. Since the FDA began its program of monitoring complaints about adverse reactions to food ingredients, 80% of the complaints concern aspartame.[1]

The confusion does not stop there. In the late1970s, Nathan Pritikin essentially changed the way we thought about our diets by promoting a low-fat, high-carbohydrate menu. At 41 years of age, Nathan had been diagnosed with arteriosclerosis and high cholesterol. He used dietary measures to correct his condition and wrote the best-selling book, *The Pritikin Program for Diet and Exercise*. About the same time, Herman Tarnower offered a diet plan for health in his book, *The Complete Scarsdale Medical Diet*. It praises the benefits of a low-fat, low-carbohydrate intake, leaving one to consume large amounts of protein. Add Barry Spears and *The Zone* to the mix. In the book, he informs us that the over-consumption of carbohydrates is a leading cause of our health problems.

Jared Fogle, the spokesman for Subway, lost 245 pounds in one year by eating a six-inch turkey sub for lunch, a 12-inch veggie sub for dinner, and exercising regularly. That's a lot of bread and a lot of carbohydrates yet he managed to lose weight. Seems like his plan of decreasing fat and increasing exercise worked quite well. If you are not sufficiently confused by now, let's toss in a healthy dose of the Atkins diet (low carbohydrates), the South Beach diet (right carbs and right fats), the Mediterranean diet (proclaiming the benefits of olive oil and grain), and the Okinawa diet (decrease caloric intake, increase energy expenditure, and consume the right kinds of food.) This could also be called the common sense diet. More information, more advice, more confusion.

Before 2005, if we were to follow the recommendations of the United States Department of Agriculture's food pyramid, you would have been consuming 6 to11 servings of bread, cereal, rice, and pasta each day. That contradicts the recommendation prescribed by *Dr. Atkin's New Diet Revolution*, *The South Beach Diet*, and *The Zone*. The old food pyramid limited the use of oils but we are now learning about the importance of the essential fatty acids found in foods such as salmon, nuts, and olive oil. How can so many experts have such differing opinions?

What about the carbohydrates, proteins, and fats we are cautioned against? Which ones are harmful and which ones are beneficial? Do not forget the axiom, "balance in everything." *The Zone* warns against eating large amounts of carrots which are chock-full of carbohydrates, whereas Scarsdale advises dieters to eat as many carrots between meals as they like. Although *The Zone* certainly holds merit when we consider the massive amounts of processed carbohydrates we eat, starting with a breakfast filled with cereal, toast, bagels, muffins, Danish pastry, or doughnuts, continuing through lunch with a more bread in a sandwich or hamburger bun, chips or French fries, and right through a dinner with more bread, pasta, potatoes, or rice. Maybe dinner was pizza and beer. Dining out at a restaurant will bring the obligatory basket of bread to the table even before the order is placed. Toss in dessert or a late night snack, perhaps a piece of pie, cake, pretzels, or a granola bar and the result is a carbohydrate overload. However, when diet plans report that the carbohydrates in bananas, carrots, cranberries, and sweet potatoes can be abusive to waistlines, I have to question that. The attention given to avoiding carbohydrates is now beyond the reaches of common sense in that multivitamins, popular soda and steak sauce are currently advertised as carbohydrate friendly. Please, enough of this nonsense. We must look at the Big Picture. We need not shun all carbohydrates but rather should avoid the overconsumption of processed carbohydrates. Think about that for a minute. Are we to believe that bananas, carrots, cranberries, and sweet potatoes are merely a storehouse of carbohydrates with nothing else to offer? Is an egg nothing but a repository for cholesterol?

Bananas are filled with potassium, vitamin C, magnesium, fiber, vitamins B1, B2, and B6. They are also low in sodium. The controversial carrot provides folic acid, magnesium, vitamin B6, thiamin, vitamin C, and beta carotene. The sweet potato also offers beta carotene, copper, vitamin C, and fiber. Cranberries are known for their ability to keep the urinary tract clean. They are an excellent antioxidant, are full of flavinoids, potassium, calcium and vitamin C; all nutrients essential to life because they keep us vital and provide the energy needed to get up each day and enjoy the world. They keep the immune system in prime working condition. These vitamins, minerals, and other cofactors provide the foundation for life. Without them, we die. Try not eating and see how long you last.

What about that poor misunderstood egg mentioned earlier? The nearsighted though is that there is cholesterol in the egg but there is also lecithin, a natural fat emulsifier. Lecithin enables cholesterol and other fats to be broken down, utilized, and then removed from the body. It protects us from cardiovascular disease and improves brain function. Cell membranes are largely composed of lecithin which allows the passage of nutrients into and out of the cell. Along with lecithin, the egg provides protein in the form of all eight essential amino acids, calcium, zinc, iron, vitamins A, E, K, B12, riboflavin, and folic acid. Those who have tried to convince us that the egg is bad for our diets because of its cholesterol do not have an understanding of the whole being greater than the sum of its parts.

A new, revolutionary, breakthrough diet emerges every year or so which allows these nutrition experts to oppose and refute each other. We need to put these diet fads into perspective. There is an underlying theme to fad diets. Though these diets may appear to have a different slant to their external packaging, they are all very similar in content: eat real whole foods, stop snacking on processed junk food, and increase the level of exercise. It is that simple. Carbohydrates, proteins and fats need to be in balance. Reducing or eliminating one can create some quick, short-term results but ignoring the body's request for balance will create some long-term problems. Diets will be successful if they extol the virtues of eating real live food which has sprung forth from the ground and not created in a factory. Diets will create lasting change if they praise the value of exercise as well as clean water. People will be healthier if life styles and diet choices are laced with a dose of common sense.

"We can either change the complexities of life... or we develop ways that enable us to cope more efficiently."
Herbert Benson

Do you think the American Medical Association can help you answer your health care concerns? Think again. If our scientific-medical community reflects the standard of health care, why does the infant mortality rate in this country rank 38th in the world?[2] There are over three dozen countries, many of which are underdeveloped, whose children are surviving infancy and living longer and healthier lives than our own children. This statistic tells me that our ruling body of health care, the AMA, by no means owns all the answers on how to obtain optimum health and therefore has no right playing the role of health care dictator.

Some yellow pages of phone books highlight the physicians section a different color. What makes physicians more important than auto mechanics? Try to make a living without your car. I want to make one thing very clear. There are no such things as experts. Someone may be more skilled at a task and someone may have more education in a particular arena, but there are no experts. No one person knows everything there is to know about one topic. No one person, or group of people, is more important than another. Modern medicine has tried to convince us otherwise. They have promoted themselves to that very position of expertise. This so-called expertise, however, is limited by one's own perspective, education, and bias.

The AMA is bound by decades of self-promoting dogma and has tried in vain to conceal any contrary point of view concerning health. Conspiring through the Committee on Quackery, which found its inception in 1963, the AMA began a campaign to contain and eliminate any practice that competed with the established medical industry.[1]

Among those attacked with slanderous barbs were chiropractors, naturopaths, homeopathy, those who promoted the use of vitamins and herbs, and alternative cancer therapies. In 1975, this Committee on Quackery and its illegal activities were exposed to the public. By 1987, Judge Susan Getzendanner, United States District Judge for the Northern District of Illinois, ruled that the AMA's conduct constituted a conspiracy to contain and eliminate the chiropractic profession and was in violation of Section 1 of the Sherman Act. The AMA was forced to admit to the lawlessness of its conduct and to publish the court's findings in *The Journal of American Medical Association*.

Though the Committee on Quackery was disbanded and the AMA paid over $50,000,000 in fines and court fees the blatant discrimination continues. Medicare will reimburse a medical doctor for an exam and x-rays. It will not pay a chiropractor for the same services. In the rare chance that a hospital exists with a chiropractor on staff, it would be akin to finding a needle in a haystack. And that chiropractor's scope of practice

---

[1] George Thomas Kurian, Illustrated Book of World Rankings, (Armonk, NY: Sharpe Reference, 2001) p. 309

will be severely limited. Acupuncture in a hospital setting is supplied by medical doctors who received their training at a seminar not in an accredited acupuncture college. We can tell our medical doctor that we are going to try chelation therapy and then note the response. We can advise our pediatrician that we do not want to expose our newborn baby to the inherent dangers in vaccines and then sit back and listen to the diatribe. We can relate to our oncologist that we have investigated the Hoxey clinic in Mexico and opt for treatment there instead of poisoning our body with chemotherapy and radiation. We will be assured to hear the words *insanity*, *ludicrous*, *asinine*, and *absurd*.

Because of this reluctance to accept other fields of health care, the majority of the population may never know how effective chiropractic care is in relieving a child from the grip of chronic ear infections. The masses will never understand the relationship between a misaligned atlas (the first bone in the neck) and its effect on congesting the Eustachian tube. After a hard rain, how easy is it for the rain water to drain into the sewers if the grates along the curbs are covered with debris? In both cases, when the obstruction is removed, the fluid drains properly. It is that simple. Children do not need to be strung out on round after round of failed antibiotic treatments. Children do not need ear tubes to create a new drainage pathway when they have their own. They merely need their God-given drainage system to become unobstructed. Then fluid will drain naturally, perfectly, just as it was designed to.

Our citizens may never know that there is a cure for everything from the common cold to cancer and it is found in the foods we eat. Though this information is available, it is suppressed and never reaches the same level of media attention as other medical and pharmaceutical information does.

Another startling piece of information that is kept from the public is that iatrogenesis, doctor-caused illness, is **the leading cause of death** in the country! Medicine, the very institution that is in charge of our health, is the number one cause of death in the United States. That ranks doctors ahead of death caused by motor vehicle accidents, lung cancer, cardiovascular disease, and AIDS. A comprehensive, independent research of peer reviewed scientific journals was completed by Gary Null, Ph.D., and others. This culminated in the article titled "Death by Medicine," published in the March 2004 edition of *Life Extension* magazine. Every charge or indictment against the AMA is supported and validated by referenced citations. The article states that 2.2 million people in hospitals every year have adverse reactions to prescribed medication. There are 7.5 million unnecessary medical and surgical procedures performed annually. Unnecessary hospitalization number nearly 9 million per year. If our stocks performed that poorly we would dump them. If our car ran that crappy we would trade it in. If a CEO of a company performed with these kinds of results the CEO would be fired (Theoretically anyway. In today's political climate, it seems poor leadership is rewarded.) And medical doctors want us to believe they are the experts on health care? Get real.

The crushing statistic cited in "Death by Medicine" is that conventional medicine is responsible for 783,936 deaths per year! Let's put that number into perspective, shall we? When just one airliner crashes, the story is headline news. The tragic accident is broadcast throughout the country in every form of media we know of. To reach the staggering number of medical caused deaths in this country you would need 10.7 jumbo jetliners seating 200 people each to crash and kill everyone on board *every single day for a full year*! Can you imagine nearly 11 airliners crashing every day for 365 days? This is the reality of our health care system yet we still allow medical doctors to dictate the necessity and protocol of care. This is an atrocity and medicine needs to be held accountable for its actions.

"Doctors pour drugs of which they know little, to cure disease of which they know less, into humans of whom they know nothing."
Voltaire

Before you finish this book, maybe the FDA will step in and help sort out the confusion. Sorry, I didn't mean to get your hopes up. Policies are created and disseminated with self-reliance in mind. Why else would vaccines be forced upon the population through intimidation and bold disrespect for our personal freedom to choose? Why has the FDA approved nonfoods such as Aspartame and MSG (which can create nervous disorders), Olestra (which brings on bouts of anal leakage), and margarine (which clogs your liver with hydrogenated fats)? Genetically altered foods no longer carry Mother Nature's design of perfection. Bovine Growth Hormones are given to the dairy cows to stimulate milk production. Why is this even needed? Have we ever had a milk shortage in this country? Do we humans need to be infected with secondary bovine growth hormones? Must our foods be preserved with cancer-causing sodium nitrates? None of these altered products have any health benefits associated with them. These non-foods have only succeeded in altering nature's already perfected foods in such a way as to benefit food-processing companies.

Have you noticed, with reference to a nutritional declaration, the disclaimer on your bottle of supplements or on the pamphlet from your herbal and vitamin store that reads, "This statement has not been evaluated by the Food and Drug Administration"? Or maybe you have seen the statement on your carton of milk declaring bovine growth hormones will cause no harm. The FDA does not have a clean record when it comes to declaring the safety of a product. Remember the grotesque birth defects related to thalidomide? How about something as seemingly innocent as a simple food coloring like yellow #5 causing rashes or red dye #2 causing tumors? The Delcon Shield and silicone breast implants have scarred generations of women. Saccharine, agent orange, asbestos, and Fen Phen were all allowed to create havoc amongst our citizens until public pressure became too great for the manufacturers of these products and the politicians who allowed their use. DES, a synthetic estrogen used in the 1950s to prevent miscarriages, created a generation of sons and daughters who suffered with incidences of infertility, reproductive hormone disorders, and cancer.

Other regulating agencies such as the Environmental Protection Agency are not all-knowing either. Some of you may remember the propaganda that was prevalent in the 1960s surrounding the safety of the pesticide DDT. A documentary that aired on public television focused on Rachel Carson, author of *A Silent Spring*. The documentary told about her fight to expose the dangers of DDT. One clip showed a darling family sitting at a picnic table eating their sandwiches all the while a truck drove by covering them with the poisonous, misting powder. The family continued to chew on their lunches with smiles on their faces. The truth concerning DDT is now known and nobody in their right mind would allow that to happen today. The EPA and FDA continue to allow poisons into our lives yet when I prescribe kelp supplements for a patient with thyroid dysfunction, I must use the disclaimer "these products are not designed to diagnose, treat, cure, or prevent disease."

Contrary to popular belief, the politicians that make up our government are not looking out for our best interest either, regardless of rhetoric and propaganda. For example, if mandatory seatbelt laws are enforced claiming seat belts save lives, why do more than half of the states allow adult motorcycle riders to take to the streets without wearing helmets? The issue then has nothing to do with safety, does it? The hypocrisy is alarming. Those who make the rules that claim to promote our safety are not all-knowing and their loyalties bend to special-interest groups like blades of grass in the wind. Common sense, instinct, and intuition have been replaced with a lust for power, greed, control, and the commerce of medicine. All those who think they are experts need to think again.

"How many ears must one man have before he can hear people cry?"
Bob Dylan

CHAPTER TWO

INTRODUCING THE MEDICINE MAN

"Peace comes within the souls of men when they realize their relationship, their oneness, with the universe and all its power and when they realize that at the center of this universe dwells Wankan Tanka,(The Great Spirit) and that this center is really everywhere. It is within each of us."
Black Elk

I grew up in a middle class white family in a middle class small town in New Hampshire. I do not believe my childhood was any different than that of most kids in my social and economic position. I was fortunate enough to have a bicycle, my own bedroom, three meals a day and four brothers to play with. Every summer the family would all congregate in the big back yard and help erect the swimming pool. I had a baseball card collection, hockey skates, and a mom who loved to kiss and hug her children. I spent my allowance on Spiderman comic books. My father took us camping and I was lucky enough to experience the magic of Disneyland. Our house was fitted with a UHF television antenna (in a time before cable was available) so I would be able to watch Bobby Orr and the Boston Bruins win a few Stanley Cups. I achieved good grades in school and did not have to struggle to make a name for myself as my oldest brother Scott had already paved the way. Being the little brother of the "big man on campus" allowed me the luxury of popularity by osmosis. I would say, for the most part, I had it pretty easy.

As much as my outside life seemed to be normal, my thoughts were not. I saw the world differently from that which was defined as normal. My mind was constantly filled with "what ifs" and "how comes." I did not always accept the explanations of my elders without reworking their information through different possibilities. There was always a part of me that questioned the norm. For example, while the masses were preaching the psychologically scarring effects of divorce on young children, I was, as a child of divorce myself, exalting in the fact that I received two birthday parties. I also was privileged to partake in two Christmases each year. After unwrapping Christmas presents with my mother and stepfather, my brothers and I would be shuffled off to repeat the same process with my father and stepmother. Hey, divorce was not all that bad. I would receive twice as many gifts!

Another example of my fledgling thinking was exposed one afternoon during our high school soccer practice. I noticed a characteristic developing among our more skilled players. When they would take practice shots on the goalie, it seemed that a vast majority of the shots were projected directly at the goalie. They were definitely powerful shots, but they did not end up in the back of the net where it counts. The goalie was not being worked out or tested very well. I spoke up and questioned their tactics. Instead of trying to blast the ball through the goalie and prove who was the most powerful, wouldn't it be to the team's advantage to develop a sense of accuracy with the shot. If you kick the ball at an unguarded part of the net, then power becomes a secondary issue. The great debate had been started: accuracy vs. sack. (That's locker room talk for the warehouse of testosterone that creates power.) The resistance I had to face from that statement was disproportionate to its innate logic: Shoot the ball where the goalie isn't standing. Why was that so hard to understand? The simple point was missed by my teammate's pubescent egos and of course they continued to shoot the ball with plenty of sack, directly at the goalie.

Several events in my childhood have undoubtedly helped to take these thoughts and mold my perception of life. They have left an indelible impression upon my understanding of the natural and spiritual processes that magically come together and form the universe we occupy. One of these events was when my mother took me to see the only chiropractor in our little town. I had wrecked up my back after taking a hard fall in one of our soccer games. As my mother was getting her chiropractic adjustment, I patiently waited in the reception room. I picked up one of the brochures from the table and began to read it. The front of the brochure said, "Don't Be an Aspirinaholic." At first, I thought this was just an interesting play on words. Comparing alcohol's addictive capacity to aspirin's seemed to be quite a stretch. How could anyone become addicted to aspirin?

The brochure went on to explain that pain is not the problem. Pain is merely a symptom of an underlying problem. By popping aspirin, (this was in a time when aspirin was the only choice for pain relief) we have not addressed the *cause* of the pain. We have only succeeded in masking the symptom of pain. This is the same as placing a sponge under the leaking faucet to stop the dripping noise: we no longer hear the spatter of the leaking drops but the leak is still there.

The aspirin itself was not the addictive quality. The act of covering up symptoms with drug after drug was the habit that could not be broken. Does it make sense to chase symptoms with drugs or to confront the cause of the symptom itself? By eliminating the cause of the pain we have not only addressed the symptoms but more importantly the origin of the symptoms. This simple but powerful concept changed my thinking to such a degree I was left completely dumbfounded. This idea made perfect sense to me. Why couldn't other people understand this point of view?

My mind immediately expanded on that thought and I questioned all forms of pharmaceuticals, not just aspirin. Aspirin became a metaphor for the entire drug industry. Blood pressure medicine can alter our blood pressure but does nothing to address the reason our blood pressure was high to begin with. Stop the medication and we still have high blood pressure. Cortisone injections can help relieve inflammation but once the cortisone is cleared from the body the cause of the inflammation still prevails. Cancer drugs, radiation, and surgery may eliminate cancerous cells but they fail to answer why the person developed cancer in the first place. Surgically removing polyps or hemorrhoids does not answer why they formed to begin with.

After some 150 years of medicine and chemicals defining our health care system, medical doctors are still masking symptom after symptom with drug after drug. I still do not see any attempt by the American Medical Association or any research body to address the *cause* of certain illnesses. The grave exception is that of chasing after some elusive secret in our genetic code. They may believe they are looking for the cause of disease by delving into the tiniest, remotest corners of the DNA strand but they are neglecting the obvious. In their quest to create life through genetic manipulation, science has forgotten how to support the already perfect life form that we inherited from our Creator. Does science really believe God makes junk? Does the medical community really think they are smarter than God? Instead of intervening in the natural process of life by introducing toxic chemicals and surgically removing vital body parts, why don't doctors focus on supporting and nurturing the body's systems with life sustaining food, oxygen, and water? Why haven't doctors, who study the same anatomy and physiology books as we chiropractors' accepted the fact that stress in the nervous system can influence the health of our tissues? Why hasn't science investigated these basics of life with the same intensity used in searching for answers supposedly hidden in the strands of DNA?

I recently taught a neuroanatomy class at a local

college. I had no sooner finished lecturing about the balance of sodium and potassium needed for cellular communication when a student raised her hand. She asked, "So too much sodium in your diet can throw off this balance and then the cells can't work properly?" Another student then chimed in, "Not only would that but the same problems exist if you did not have enough potassium, right?" Absolutely, emphatically 100% correct! How come 20-year-old college students can see this basic cellular relationship and correlate its dysfunction to a simple nutritional equation but scientific research cannot? Compare the number of commercials on television that promote arthritis medicine to those commercials advertising the health benefits of raw apple cider vinegar.

Another event in my childhood that inevitably helped mold my philosophical outlook was the fact that for a period of time my mother and stepfather hosted Bible study at our house once a week. My bedroom was directly above the sitting room where these get-togethers took place. The house I grew up in was an old farmhouse that had small trap doors in the upstairs flooring to let the heat from the wood stove below circulate through the other rooms. This also allowed me the perfect opportunity to eavesdrop and I became familiar with their interpretations of the biblical stories in this way.

However, when it comes to the interpretation of an event, whose interpretation do we give credence to? If we choose to see spirituality through Christian eyes, we are then confronted with choosing a sect. Will our Christian beliefs align with one of the many Baptist or Lutheran branches, Orthodox or Roman Catholic, Presbyterian, Methodist, Protestant, Seventh Day Adventist, Pentecostal, or Jehovah's Witnesses? Perhaps we feel more comfortable with the biblical interpretations of Christian Science, Unitarianism, or Episcopalian dogma. When it came to one God one religion I couldn't figure out which one Christianity was speaking of. Again, questions would emerge.

When I heard the creation story, I wondered why science and religion argued so intensely over how the beginning of this world came about. Isn't the story of creation the same as the Big Bang theory? It is just told in a different language. The Bible version is more poetic and speaks in spiritual tones while the Big Bang theory creates our world in the language of science. In both cases, the world as we know it was created from nothing. The Bible's version took seven days and the scientific version took millions of years. What if a million years as seen by linear-thinking humans were but a blink of an eye to a God that has no beginning and no end? In 2 Peter 3:8 it even states, "Be not ignorant of this one thing, that one day is with the Lord as a thousand years, and a thousand years as one day." Sounds like God does not have a time reference. In the beginning, God created heaven and earth. That must have made a pretty big bang.

"Great spirits have always experienced violent opposition from mediocre minds"
Albert Einstein

Christians are taught that God made man in his own image. Does that mean man is a mirror image of God himself or does that simply mean that the image itself belonged to God? Does the emphasis on "image" mean that of a physical representation of the original or is it instead the nonphysical picture in the mind that merely belonged to God? I can imagine a fancy sports car. This is my own image. The image belongs to me but the sports car is not a mirror image of me. If it was just the image of man that belonged to God then God may not look anything like us. God just may very well be in yet a completely different form. If God created us in his own image, it does not mean we have to look like

God but rather the image of us itself belonged to God. It all depends on how one decides to define the words and their meanings. Lest we forget, that is only one concern in translating the English version of the scriptures. How many words were misrepresented in translating spiritual text from their original languages? If one word can draw up this much confusion as to the meaning of a statement, what can be said for the entire interpretation of any religious work?

I could not accept the story of Noah as blind faith either. First of all, the 2004 publication of the Encyclopedia Americana states there are over 2,700 species of snakes in the world and there are over 100,000 different kinds of butterflies and moths. I could not believe that one man could span the globe and collect two of every creature with these kinds of massive numbers confronting him. Second, some animals are indigenous to certain climates. One would have to travel to the far reaches of the ice caps to acquire penguins and polar bears. Did Noah visit Australia for a kangaroo and then skip to Colorado to trap some bald eagles? It would take several lifetimes in this era of technology to acquire such a menagerie never mind completing the tasks without the aid of modern tools.

Can you imagine how much food it would take to feed all these animals for forty days and forty nights? With 5,400 snakes to feed (one male and one female for each different species of snake) at one mouse per week, times 4.5 weeks, Noah and his family need 243,000 mice just to feed these snakes. Do you see how this feeding dilemma can quickly grow out of control? What would Noah need to keep 243,000 mice alive? How did he keep the birds from eating the worms? Why didn't the lions attack the zebras? How much eucalyptus does a Koala bear eat in forty days?

Maybe the stories in the Bible are not meant to be taken literally. Maybe they are part mythology, part analogy, part faith-based life lessons, and part spiritual mystery. Other religions accept their mythology as part of the basis for their particular religion. Christian fundamentalists completely disavow mythology and want us to accept the word of the Bible as true fact. However, as I familiarized myself with Revelation I was confronted with "horses with lion's heads breathing smoke, fire and sulfur, with tails of serpents unleashing their wrath." That kind of description just reeks of mythology.

As I listened to these Bible groups discussing their faith, I found it ironic that Christian families would indulge in the pagan rituals concerning the Easter Bunny. Years later I actually met a pastor of a church who would perform his Easter sermon to his congregation and then drive off to the mall to dress up in the Easter Bunny costume and pass out candy to the children. Can anyone say "conflict of interest?" How can Christians justify the yearly participation of decorating a Christmas tree? This evergreen may be named in accord with their holy holiday but the symbolism has pagan roots. I am not defaming Christianity as a religion. I am merely pointing out discrepancies I noticed as a young eavesdropping child. If I had been raised in an Islamic family, I would be relating my experiences through Islamic eyes.

"If a man does not keep pace with his companions, perhaps it is because he hears a different drummer. Let him step to the music which he hears, however measured or far away."
Henry David Thoreau

The point I am trying to make here is that I came to realize that I could not accept information as undeniable fact just because some authority figure deemed it so. This did not exclusively pertain to religion. Did George Washington really chop down a cherry tree and confess to his father of his transgression or is that a nice way to teach children not to lie? How much of what we hear is truth and how much is exaggerated through legend? Does repeating a story over and over again allow the reality to grow beyond its own believability yet we still continue to believe it?

As soon as I was old enough to understand the nature of competitive sports I could not understand how a professional football team could get away with calling themselves the Redskins. That is a derogatory name with no way to justify its use. I do not see any professional teams calling themselves the Columbus Crackers or the Williamsburg Wetbacks. Where are the Baltimore Blackies and the Seattle Slant Eyes? Sound a little racist? So does Redskin. How many teams named Warriors have ever sported a logo other than an American Indian? Are the indigenous people of this continent the only people ever to go to war? Why aren't there any Warrior teams with jerseys sporting emblems of World War II veterans? They were warriors. Napoleon was a warrior as was Julius Caesar but in the sporting arenas across this country only American Indians are symbolic of warriors.

History taught us about the atrocities committed by Adolf Hitler and World War II Germany. We learned about the forced relocation of Jews into ghettos. Families were separated and brutality was the norm. We read stories of the millions of Jews that were tortured, experimented on, raped, murdered, and burned in ovens. What did school teach us concerning the plight of the American Indian? We learned about their generosity toward the pilgrims and the founding of Thanksgiving. We learned about how Sacagawea helped Lewis and Clark through the wilderness of the western frontier. The impression implanted in us as children was that the American Indians were glad to see us and, for the most part, were willing to give up their land for us. When in truth, their story is no different than that of the Jewish people of the 1940s. Millions of Native Americans were murdered, raped, and forced into slavery. Their land was stolen and they were brutally treated. Their culture was destroyed as we fed them a steady diet of small pox and alcohol. Their sacred buffalo was slaughtered by the millions. Why was it all right to point the finger at Hitler's treatment of Jews to demonstrate evil but not do the same to the United States government and their treatment of the American Indian?

Politics did not escape my analytical criticism. In school, we learned about our founding fathers and the writing of the Declaration of Independence which proclaimed that all men are created equal. Yet they somehow found justification for the slave trade as well as the aforementioned annihilating of millions of native people to quench their own greed for conquest. Women had no rights either. They could not own land and could not vote. Women were as much a piece of property as the slaves were. That did not seem very equal to me. I guess when the founding fathers wrote the word "men" in the Declaration, they meant only white men of European descent.

I do not claim to be the only one who owns these points of view. You, too, may have questioned some of these very same ideas. However, my mind was revolving around these thoughts long before any signs of puberty. I had no one to share them with. Other kids my age were experimenting with Spin the Bottle or riding their bicycles in the park while I was wondering what a bumper sticker with the letters MIA and POW meant. When I questioned a traditional paradigm, adults would remind me that I thought too much. I was told "that's just the way it is" or "just because." My all-time least favorite response was the inevitable, "Because I said so. That's why."

Why do I continue on this pursuit for answers, for truth? Why do I debate the routines of the medical establishment? Why do I harbor such a desire to question everything? Examine the word *question* closely. When you break the word apart, you will find an "ion" and a "quest." A question then becomes a charged particle on a journey. I am that charged particle on that journey. My life is the symbolic question. My charged mission is a quest to find the truth. Being involved in the field of health care and also being involved in the care of planet Earth, I want to know what forces come together to create man and life and how can we keep these forces running properly and in harmony with each other.

I want to know how health care has metastasized into disease care. I want to know why we have exchanged the essentials of life; oxygen, nutrition, water, exercise, and common sense for unnecessary surgeries and chemically altering our bodies with synthetic, toxic pharmaceuticals. I want to know why some medical doctors refuse to acknowledge and refer their patients to other healing arts if the welfare of their patients is the primary goal. I want to know where in time man ever, for one second, began to think he was smarter than the Universal Intelligence (God has a thousand names) that gave us all life.

"The struggle with most people is largely one of man against himself, between abnormal darkness of ignorance and natural light of understanding."
B. J. Palmer

I am indeed an ion on a quest to regenerate hope and faith in the knowledge that the powers that made the body heal the body. I am alive with the understanding that the innate wisdom that created us from one sperm and one egg did not desert us at birth and that the same infinite miracle that began our existence is still inside us working to keep us alive. I want to rekindle the knowledge that the healing power of our body does not stop at fighting off a cold or mending a scraped knee. That very same energy is inside us this very second, keeping us safe from all those forces that create illness and debilitating disease. The immune system and our endowed right to health do not take a vacation after we are born. They do not leave us helpless, alone in a field surrounded by wolves. Our ability to heal is 100% functional, adaptable, and programmable. The healing of a broken bone is no different than that of the healing of a malignant tumor. Of course there are specialized physiological functions for each process but the commitment and desire of our body to heal is constant, 100% of the time, every second of every day.

My learning and questioning did not end with the onset of adulthood. In fact, it continues to drive me every day. Listen to the television ads today promoting pharmaceuticals. They are some of the best entertainment on TV. The list of side effects takes longer to scroll through than the commercial itself. It is a great feeling to relieve the symptoms of allergies but now our liver and both kidneys are damaged, our skin itches, hemorrhoids have developed, and we have developed chronic headaches. But by God our breathing is easier. With this blatant attack of our common sense, we are still cautioned to seek the advice of our medical doctors who dispense these pharmaceuticals at will. What I see here is a dose of self-imposed job security by the AMA. The more drugs they dispense, the more sick people they have to watch over.

The major problem with our system of health care is caused by the difference between how nature truly operates and how man thinks nature should operate. We have been programmed through years of medical-political special interest groups to believe that once we have become stricken with disease we must seek the advice of a doctor if we are to ever re-establish a state of health. Basic knowledge of life, understanding those very elements and energies that create and sustain life, have been reconstructed and perverted into empirical theories that have led us all to live in a world of misperception. Science is so busy analyzing the intricate complexities of life that they have failed to realize that life does not need a babysitter.

People find it easier to blame doctors for not finding a miracle cure than to take personal responsibility and change poor lifestyle choices. If we give the body what it needs to survive it will in turn do its job by providing us with a lifetime of health. If we instead pollute it with toxic chemicals, either in the form of pharmaceuticals, food additives and preservatives, cigarettes, recreational drugs, or other man-made environmental pollution, we will reap what we sow. Staying healthy is not a big mystery that is waiting to be unraveled. It is a physiological scaffold built into the very creation of life. Life and health always was, is, and ever shall be. There is no big secret here. There is no Pandora's Box, no genie in a bottle, and no fountain of youth. There's just some common sense and the application of such within the boundaries of perfection that is the creation of life.

"For things to reveal themselves to us, we need to be ready to abandon our views about them."
Thich Nhat Hanh

CHAPTER THREE

WHO TOLD YOU THAT AND WHY DO YOU BELIEVE THEM?

"We never know how far reaching something we may think, say, or do today will affect the lives of millions tomorrow."
B. J. Palmer

The world is not as it appears. The world is as we *think* it appears. You are participating in a paradigm of misperception, and it is that misperception that keeps you locked into your state of illness or disease. Our sense of reality does not define our thoughts about life. Our thoughts about life define our reality. Just what does all that mumbo-jumbo mean anyway? Sounds like a bunch of hocus-pocus psychobabble doesn't it? Am I actually going to try to convince you that your belief system is the reason you are sick? Yes I am! Am I going to reassure you that your genes are not to blame for your problems? Absolutely! Am I going to try to help you understand that the steps you must take to overcome your health care issues can be as easy as learning how to ride a bicycle? Definitely!

If your thoughts define your world, then they must define your health as well. Now that I have your attention, go back and read the first five sentences of the last paragraph one more time. Here's what I mean. Consider something as obvious as the President of the United States. He is the same person no matter who describes him. As our elected leader, the president is a living symbol of the nation. His physical routine is identical to all those who care to examine it. He creates policy that he believes will benefit the country. He visits foreign countries as a diplomat and tries to spread the agenda of democracy. His decisions ultimately affect not only Americans but the whole world as well. Every president has the opportunity to leave a legacy of his achievements. Each term has the potential to be etched with scandal. What are your thoughts and how do you define the current administration? Past administrations? What if the current president belonged to a different party? Would your level of appreciation change? You can ask ten people on the street to describe the president and rate his performance and you will get ten different answers.

Jimmy Carter wanted to boycott the Olympics. Should politics be part of the Olympics? Was that a good decision or was that a bad one? How do you assimilate that action? Ronald Reagan is given credit for winning the Cold War and having the communist East Germans tear down the Berlin Wall. Was he really responsible for that act or was it inevitable that the wall would come down due to changes in world opinion? Was he just in the right place at the right time? When you hear the words "weapons of mass destruction" what feeling do they generate in you? How is it that the facts surrounding one event can be manipulated to create distinctively different versions of the exact same story? The reality of the presidency does not define our thoughts, or we would all think the same way about the president. One person, one act, one thought. Your thoughts define the character of the president. He is the same man who by performing one sole act can be defined differently. You see the president and the rest of the world, including your health, through your thoughts about how you think things are. So who told you to think the way you do and why did you believe them? Is your way of thinking the only way to think?

Taking a very brief tour through history can help us understand the answer to that question. The ancient Greeks lived in a world of polytheism. Their art, science, and philosophy, their entire culture, all reflected this belief in a universe controlled by many gods. They lived their lives with the conviction that the gods could at any time with the wave of their hand create floods, famine, and death, or conversely create a great harvest, warm summer, and even allow for a man and a woman to conceive. It was the job of the mortals to live life in accordance with the divine laws set forth by these gods. Failing to do so could evoke the god's wrath upon the people and the land. This definition of reality was strong enough to produce classic philosophy by Socrates, Plato, and Aristotle. Pythagoras created mathematical theories while participating in this belief system. Myron was so inspired to sculpt his famous discus thrower, Discobolus. By the end of the Roman Empire the belief in a one god world became the predominant paradigm. Christianity took over as the standard-bearer and gained secular authority. This change in conviction created quite a struggle amongst the cultures as civilization propelled through the Inquisition, the Crusades, and the Dark Ages. From this monotheistic paradigm, we came to marvel at the religious works of Bellini's *Madonna and Child* and *Lamentation Over the Body of Christ*. Botticelli was inspired to create the *Adoration of the Magi* as well as the *Temptation of Christ*. Michelangelo painted his classic frescoes on the ceiling of the Sistine Chapel. These men were motivated to greatness by believing in this particular world paradigm. We were given some powerfully spiritual teachings dictated through Jesus Christ. Though the many sects within Christianity may define Jesus' teachings differently, we were told to love our neighbor as ourselves and we were taught that forgiveness is the ultimate sacrifice.

      The biblical, Christian world view, like other world views, gave way to yet another. The scientific world view that followed was propelled to the forefront of mainstream thought by Rene Descartes, Isaac Newton, Francis Bacon, Galileo and others. These men indoctrinated us into the belief that the world and everything on it operated like a machine and did not require God to control it. The functions of the world could be reduced to simple mathematical equations.

The planet's orbital rotations became a product of math, not God. The arc of an object thrown through the air was directed by force, gravity, and acceleration. The velocity of a falling object could be determined and duplicated over and over again.

The world became one that was not alive with spirit but was mechanical and analytical. Physics as a branch of science developed and the nature and properties of matter and energy could be predicted mathematically. No longer were events thought of as part of God's master plan. The mysterious events in nature lost favor. The phenomena of time, for example, was pulled from nature and captured in a mechanical clock. No longer dictated by God, the clock took the place of the different seasons and the orbits of the planets as the favorite time piece. The universe was no longer awe inspiring. Spirit was stripped from the human body as well and we were left with a heart that pumped blood, muscles that created motion, and lungs that passed our breath to our body. Ballistic curves and wave theory became the ultimate laws of the environment. Scientific theory became the dominating philosophy. Nature was no longer a secret. It could all be calculated and analyzed as pieces of the whole.

These world views changed only because the thought process that dominated at that time eventually changed. We all live on the same planet, drink the same water, feel the same thunder storms, and coexist with the same animals. We still write plays, raise families, and cheer the athlete. We still create governments, listen to music, and grow old. Earthquakes still move mountains, snow is still cold, and wars are still waged. It is the same planet. Only the thoughts about how we live and how the world operates have changed. Our perception of the world changed and that changed our sense of reality.

Man's science, art, and philosophy will penetrate through his filter of perception creating the very reality he expects. Your expectations of a person, place, thing, or idea is what gives that object life and definition. Your sense of reality is based not on what life gives you but how you interpret life's offerings.

"The voyage of discovery is not in seeking new landscape but in having new eyes."
Marcel Proust

At one time it was blasphemous to speak of a universe in which the sun was at the center. Prior to Copernicus, the religious and philosophical sense was that of an earth-based center of the solar system. Copernicus dared to defy some 1,500 years of organized religious dogma. The conviction that the earth was the center of our solar system was so concretized that his ideas were labeled heresy by the Roman Catholic Church and the Vatican banned his publications until 1822. Galileo confirmed Copernicus's discovery and he too was dealt a similar fate. He was denounced as a heretic, tried during the Spanish Inquisition, and forced to renounce his beliefs. In the 1500s, the Roman Catholic Church so believed that the planets revolved around the earth they were willing to abolish opposing opinions. Their thoughts created the world they lived in even though reality was not in line with their belief system.

Here are a few more examples of how changing your thought changes your reality. Prior to 1903 very few people considered the idea that man could fly, leaving flight to the birds. Then Orville and Wilbur Wright showed us differently. In less than 100 years of flight, we now have space shuttles orbiting the earth. Who, before that historic day at Kitty Hawk, would have believed man could fly? The Wright brothers' belief, their thought process, created a change in our perception of reality. The world has become smaller because we can now travels hundreds of miles in a fraction of the time that it used to take. The ability to fly has always been a part of reality. It took a change in thought to create a tangible expression of that ability. The thought process changed our reality.

Into the 1950s, many women in the United States were raised to believe that it was their duty, their role in life, to find a man to marry and to have his children. The average woman did not contemplate college not to mention a career. In many cases marriage and babies were the prerequisites to societal acceptance. Try to relegate an American woman to that role today and see how far you get. Women today are as active in college as men, if not more, and they are certainly just as career oriented. Their function in life has changed dramatically. Women are no longer just baby makers but now are CEOs and world leaders. Was this change brought on because the women physically changed into some new species? Did women somehow develop more brain cells? Did they take self-esteem pills? No. Women are women, whether in 1950 or today. Same anatomy and same physiology. What changed was the paradigm that guided them. It was the thoughts concerning women's roles that changed thus allowing a new reality to develop. Our thoughts changed our view of the world.

In today's scientific realm we are changing our world view from a linear, reductionist one to one of holism defined by quantum physics. Linear thinking, in a nut shell, is the mechanical paradigm left to us by Newton, Descartes, Bacon, and Galileo. Using it, one believes that once we understand all the parts that make up the whole, we can remove the broken part, fix it, and replace it back into the model. That is to say, A+B+C+D=ABCD, or our heart + our veins and arteries + our capillaries + our blood = our cardiovascular system. If we succumb to a heart attack, science can go find and replace the broken part, in this case the clogged artery, by performing bypass surgery. They have fixed the broken piece of the equation and the whole system should operate normally once again. They can also repair broken parts by chemically altering them with pharmaceuticals. If 1+2+3+4=1234, or our hydrochloric acid and digestive enzymes + our stomach + our small intestine + our large intestine = our digestive system, we can alter the pattern of heartburn by chemically changing the "1" in the equation. Our body and our systems have been reduced to replaceable parts. This surgical-chemical, linear intervention is the driving force behind medicine.

Alas, life is not that simple and Albert Einstein proved just that with his Theory of Relativity. Physics, up until the 1940s, was the study of the interaction between matter and energy as two distinct entities. The field of quantum physics emerged from Einstein's work and proved that energy and matter are actually the same thing. Quantum physics uncovered a whole new world image. With help from Einstein the world was no longer looked upon as a machine with distinct individual parts that could be analyzed by separating them from the whole. There was no longer the ability to manipulate one piece of the equation without affecting the entirety of the equation or system. The atom, the smallest unit of matter, was found to be not a physical structure but rather an energetic influence. The physical world is comprised of electromagnetic pulses of energy that all interacted with each other on some level. Through quantum physics, the linear, reductionist equation noted earlier now took on a new shape and looked like this (see figure 1).

We cannot replace, change, or chemically alter one part without completely changing the entire structure. This is why pharmaceuticals have inherent side effects. Medicine wants a certain drug to affect only part B in the linear equation. Quantum physics says you cannot affect part B without affecting parts A, C, and D as well. A, C, and D become the side effects we experience. This new concept of electromagnetic interactions is referred to as holism. Parts of any whole cannot exist nor can they be completely understood except in relationship to the entire structure.

"A" no longer affects only "B" as in the linear equation. In this quantum physics model, "A" has an effect on all the parts of the equation including

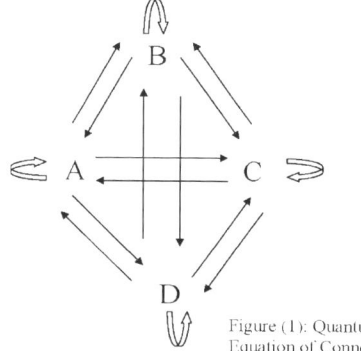

Figure (1): Quantum Physics Equation of Connectedness

itself. One part cannot be singled out and treated without influencing every other part of the system.

Working within a model of quantum physics, all matter is reduced to its electromagnetic, molecular vibration. This vibration gives off a frequency which is unique to that structure. The atoms of broccoli vibrate at a different frequency than the atoms of a lemon. Iron differs from lead because of their atomic, electromagnetic makeup and how their atoms resonant with each other. Healthy lung tissue vibrates with a molecular frequency different from that of cancerous lung tissue.

The health of our body cannot be reduced to our cholesterol levels or our blood pressure. Those are pieces of the whole body's design. Parts of any whole cannot exist and certainly cannot be understood except in relation to the whole. Quantum physics takes into consideration not only how these pieces vibrate together within the body, but also how the body reacts to the external environment. Everything from the smallest subatomic particle to the largest planet in the sky is in relationship with all other matter. Quantum physics is analogous to an orchestral performance. Hundreds of notes (vibrational frequencies) from a multitude of different instruments (heart, lungs, bowels, kidneys, muscles, hormones, etc.) all come together to create one perfectly resonating piece of music (our body.) If one musician playing one instrument hits one wrong note the whole symphony (our health) changes for the worse.

Since Einstein's discovery, all forms of science except therapeutic medicine have embraced this new concept of life and we have reaped the benefits from this realm of electromagnetic energy. We use computer chips and cell phones with untamed enthusiasm. These take our physical world and compress it into electromagnetic impulses. Fax machines take a tangible piece of paper with a message typed on its face and convert it into an electromagnetic impulse. This impulse travels through a wire (and through air if wireless) to its destination and is transformed once again into its original, physical idea. Matter is converted to its energetic blueprint and this energetic blueprint is altered once again into its material form.

Deepak Chopra is a leader in the field of mind body medicine. He is the founder of the Chopra Center for Well Being, an author of more than thirty books, and an established endocrinologist. In relation to our own health, his great work has shown us how our beliefs, thoughts, and feelings can take physical form not only in our biochemistry but also as an electromagnetic wave of energy that can affect an outcome in our physiology. He has given the power of thought a substantial scientific base.

I had a patient who had suffered a stroke several years earlier. She related to me the events leading up to her stroke listing several events of consequential magnitude. Her husband had divorced her. Her house had burned down, her son had died, and her pet dog was hit by a car. Any one of these events can be, in and of itself, too much to handle, but she was burdened with all of them within a relatively short period of time. She told me there was so much going on in her mind that she thought her head would explode. In fact, it did just that. The intensity of her thoughts resulted in an explosion in her head. The very fact that the placebo effect exists proves that something as intangible as a thought can create tangible physical change.

The x-ray machine has evolved into computerized axial tomography (CAT scans), electron-beam tomography, magnetic resonance imaging (MRI), and now total body scans. All these machines were products of learning how to manipulate the electromagnetic vibrations of our universe. These latest technologies transform our organ's vibrational frequencies into a visible working diagnosis. The total body scan can detect the differences between healthy heart tissue and diseased heart tissue because these tissues have distinctly different vibrational makeup.

Medicine will use these products of quantum physics only to diagnose abnormalities but will turn a blind eye to quantum physics when it comes to actual treatment. In regards to treatment, medicine still operates in a world of removable, replaceable parts without considering the whole structure. Instead of researching a way to re-create the electromagnetic, molecular vibration of healthy lung tissue in a cancerous lobe, they continue to use the linear equation of reductionism. Surgically removing or irradiating a part of the lung perpetuates the A+B+C+D=ABCD model. The quantum physics model would treat the person's diseased lung tissue with vibrational elements that resonate with the frequency of healthy tissue thereby restoring the lung to its energetic blueprint and promoting healthy interactions between all the systems of the body. The failure of this country's health care system resides in this very fact: medicine operates in a paradigm of yesteryear and therefore is out of touch with the current state of reality.

New world paradigms evolve through our efforts to change our pattern of thinking. Quantum physics has existed since the beginning of time but we could not appreciate its complexities until we created a thought process that could accept it. Medicine continues to drag its heels when it comes to accepting the new world paradigm. Admitting to or accepting a paradigm different than the one used by the current medical establishment would be, in their eyes, an admission of error. In reality, it is not an error. It is a change in thinking. That does not mean that the rest of us have to stick our heads in the sand as well. We have the freedom to learn, think, and consciously evolve without approval from the medical industry. We are free to accept the role of quantum physics without dissecting the Theory of Relativity. We can appreciate a world that pulses with electromagnetic energy and incorporates holism without an FDA stamp of approval.

Who told us that we have to develop Alzheimer's disease because our father had it? An outdated paradigm. Why do we believe it? Who told us that we have to fall apart when we reach the age of 50, or is it 40, or is it 30? An outdated paradigm. Why do we believe it? Do we still believe that men can't fly or that women are only good for making babies? Reality will mimic our thoughts. Changing our thoughts will change our reality.

Diseases do not just fall from the sky and hit us on the head. We do not just wake up one day with rheumatoid arthritis because our genes have all of a sudden gone bad. It is not the fault of our genes or our destiny to become sick because one outdated view of the world dictates it to be so. The new paradigm of quantum physics suggests that our genes are not programmed with self-destruct mechanisms. Self-destructive genes are the complete antithesis of life. If our genes were programmed with a design to kill us, we would cease to exist. The human experience continues because our genes are programmed with knowledge of life not death.

Now we have two world views confronting us. Which do we choose? Will we believe the one that claims that life has a built-in self-destruct mechanism that destroys its host by creating disease and premature degeneration or will we choose the one that promotes life, understands the Big Picture, and supports the idea of self-expression?

Physical matter has a life expectancy and does eventually wear out but its energetic blueprint will live on. I contend we may never know the truth as to the life expectancy of our physical matter as long as we continue to operate within the constructs of the linear equation A+B+C+D=ABCD without accepting our interconnectedness with not only ourselves but the entire planet.

A healer must understand the limitations of linear thinking. A 49-year-old woman came to my office who had recently been diagnosed with multiple sclerosis. She had experienced numbness on the left side of her face and an MRI revealed swelling in the brain stem. She also suffered from chronic sinusitis and a ringing in her left ear. The medical doctors that she consulted were locked into linear thinking; brain stem swelling of unknown origin + facial paralysis + sensory disruption = multiple sclerosis. This was not what the patient wanted to hear. When I examined her, I found a severe misalignment with her atlas, the first bone in the neck. It had shifted to the right side. The second bone in the neck, axis, was misaligned to the left side. This right-left zigzag of her cervical vertebrae was choking the neuronal centers located in her brain stem. She was given a chiropractic spinal adjustment and three days later at her follow-up appointment she was pain free.

Holistic thinking involves consideration of all parts, every aspect.

This is the age of holism as directed by the tenets of quantum physics. We may choose to remain in the old paradigm of reductionism if we like. Nobody is forcing us to accept these beliefs. We choose to do so all on our own. We may also choose to use a ten year old computer with dial-up service to surf the internet. Time changes as our thought process changes.

One day, as our thoughts expand, the limitations of reality based on quantum physics will be exposed and yet another world view will emerge. Quantum physics is not the end of our conscious thinking. It is a new beginning. Our culture mimics what our thoughts allow. If we believe that it is our destiny to grow old and suffer the ravages of arthritis, heart disease or cancer, we will. If we believe that there is a better way to maintain our health, we will find it, the same way the Wright Brothers believed we could fly and "found" the airplane. If we do not believe we can fly, we never will.

"The higher we soar, the smaller we appear to those who cannot fly."
Nietzsche

CHAPTER FOUR

WEEDING OUT THE GARDEN

"Gardens are not made by sitting in the shade"
Rudyard Kipling

As we walk through this garden of health care "expertise," it seems we are just as likely to grab a handful of weeds as we are to lay down in a bed of roses. In terms of our health care, we are receiving half-truths, hopeful expectations, personal bias, slanted research, and even out and out lies. Every time we hear about the latest research confirming the views of a certain party, please remember, somebody funded that research and wants to promote a certain viewpoint. Research will show us exactly what those paying for the research want us to see. For every article published in a peer review journal claiming any sort of analysis, there are just as many research articles debunking the exact same reference. One reason the American Indians revere the bald eagle as a highly spiritual entity is because it can soar above the clouds. In doing so, the eagle flies so high that when it looks down at the earth below, it can see both sides of the mountain. That is, there are two sides to every story. Only by understanding the two halves can you come to appreciate the whole.

The greatest heart surgeon in the world may know precisely how to perform a triple bypass operation. After the procedure has been completed, does the heart surgeon realize that he has only bypassed the symptom of the blockage (chest pain) and not addressed the cause of the blockage (maybe poor dietary choices)? The bypass surgery bypasses every factor that contributed to the condition in the first place. The surgeon has done nothing but reroute the prior condition. And what does this brilliant doctor know about the powers of vitamin E, lecithin, and garlic for removing the plaque in the arteries and keeping the blood clean within the circulatory system? Has this doctor studied the acupuncture heart meridian and know how to manipulate the energies traversing within it? Will this doctor give any validity to the Ayurvedic traditions of the bio-energetic activity of the heart chakra and its relationship to disease?

    A patient of mine, Sue, was experiencing fluttering in her heart. She was run through a battery of tests only to find everything was normal. Does this mean that she is lying about her condition? Should she wait until medicine has developed technology to diagnose her condition properly and then go back to her doctor? Her heart flutters were diagnosed and resolved with traditional Chinese medicine. Anxiety was the culprit. Through their own advancements in technology, medical science has tried in vain to dissect life in an attempt to find all the answers to immortality. The human DNA chain has been analyzed strand by strand hoping that the mysteries of life will spring forth with the enthusiasm of a genie that has finally been released from his bottle.

"Simplicity is the ultimate sophistication."
Leonardo Da Vinci

    Herein lays the folly of science. Medical science is forever trying to "one-up" Mother Nature. Mother Nature is the synthesis of life not the laboratory. Will a cloned baby have a soul like those babies born through natural conception? Will its consciousness have a separate and unique identity or will it be trapped by the original owner's past? A newborn cloned from a fifty year old's DNA will be born with fifty year old DNA, complete with all the genetic markers and life experiences of a fifty year old person. If all went well with this misguided experiment, would we only expect this clone to live for 30 or so years? Though this clone may be just a newborn, it is, after all, a copy from fifty year old DNA. How will the stimulation of a completely different upbringing interact with someone else's preprogrammed DNA?

The more science tries to dissect and analyze, the more it loses touch with the very process of life itself. Life is not one DNA strand nor is it one kind of bacteria isolated in a Petrie dish. The rhythms of our universe cannot be separated into neat little packages. We are not pieces to be conveniently labeled and put on a shelf. The seasons are not separated by days on a calendar. They blend into each other with effortless ease. Night cannot be separated from the day. When does one day start and the other stop? At dusk and dawn, sunrise and sunset, 6:00 am and 6:00 pm? Science attempts to look deeper and deeper into the minutest pieces of life expecting to find the one answer to our health problems. While science examines inwardly from without, what it needs to do is just the opposite; examine outwardly from within. The secrets to health are found in examining our relationships with all other living pieces and parts as one whole unit. It is not found in dissecting ourselves into bits and isolating them from a world filled with stimulation.

Take for example something as common as vitamin C. Everybody knows vitamin C is good for the immune system. We catch a cold and head straight for the orange juice or take extra supplements. But check the multivitamin and see how the vitamin C is supplied. Unless we are utilizing whole food supplements, we will see vitamin C listed as ascorbic acid. Once again, those so called experts have simplified the elaborate myriad of life into one element. Ascorbic acid is not vitamin C. It is only a fraction of the whole vitamin C complex. The vitamin C complex also contains bioflavonoids and rutin which help maintain vascular integrity. The vitamin C complex embodies P, K, and J factors that help blood coagulate and increase the oxygen-carrying capacity of the blood. The vitamin C complex supplies us with the enzyme tyrosinase which activates the adrenal glands. Then there is hesperidin which helps maintain the strength of the capillaries and other connective tissue. And that is only the tip of the iceberg. There may be more to the vitamin C complex that still eludes investigation than that which we know about. It is the presence of all these factors, known and unknown, that create the synergistic alchemy of vitamin C. It loses its power when we start to dismember the sum of its parts. These "experts" in charge of our health lose sight of the overall natural process, the Big Picture, when they focus on one aspect of the complexity that is called life. Yes, vitamin C is good for the immune system but that statement references a whole food complex vitamin C not processed pasteurized juice or ascorbic acid supplements.

The key to a healthy lifestyle lies in understanding Natural Law and the application of some good old fashion common sense. When I tell patients that something as simple as drinking more pure, clean water can be a factor in decreasing their discomfort, they have trouble believing me. The population has been brainwashed into believing that health can only be acquired through a medical professional and dispensed via a pharmacist. Health is not determined by our intake of antibiotics or any other pharmaceutical. It cannot be legislated through mass vaccination programs or socialized medicine. A strict regimented formula does not allow for the diversity of creation to work its magic.

The irony is that the medical community's quest for the answers to life is pulling them ever further from the very answers in which they seek. It's as if the scientific community has set up institutions to prove it has cornered the market on truth. The simple truth is that life just happens. The salmon do not need watches to tell them when it is time to swim upstream to spawn. Monarch butterflies do not require maps to find their way home from Capistrano. Summer needs not a plastic surgeon to change into autumn. Bears do not require alarm clocks to wake them from hibernation. Spiders do not have to read blueprints to create an intricate web. The brilliant uniqueness of each shiny, new snowflake is not born in a test tube. As hard as science tries, it will never turn grass into milk without a cow. It will not make an egg without a chicken.

"Animals do better by instinct than man does by reason."
Mark Twain

Jerry Lewis has helped the Muscular Dystrophy Association raise over one billion dollars since 1966. How have we benefited from all that research? Nearly four decades of spending and still no return on the investment. Don't we hear the same story every year? The answer is just around the corner. We are so close to finding a cure. All we need is just a few more dollars.

If we dropped a piece of jewelry on the floor and thought it rolled under the couch, would we spend four decades looking for it? Thirty five days? One week? How long would we crawl around with our focus under the couch before we turn around, scratch our chin, and think to look from another vantage point? With this tendency for research to delve into the tiniest, remotest, genetic structures in search of answers to diseases, they have put all their eggs into one basket. The only thing science has perfected here is a chronic case of tunnel vision.

In 1971, President Richard Nixon declared war on cancer. He vowed that science would find a cure to cancer within seven years. Appropriate funds were diverted to support the effort. Cancer is responsible for one of every four deaths in this country.[2] An estimated

---

[2] Karen Bellenir, Cancer Source Book, 4th Edition, Health Reference Series, (Detroit, MI: Omnigraphics, Inc., 2003), p. 31.

1,500 people died of cancer every day in 2002.[43] If this is a war, we are losing. Yet with all this focus on creating cancer vaccines and toxic chemical therapies, there is no interest from the FDA, American Cancer Society, Harvard Medical School, or any other research firm to investigate Laetrile or Essiac Tea as cancer therapies. The only publicity Laetrile and Essiac Tea have generated has been the sweeping, bold statement that these two treatments have been deemed not scientifically based. Laetrile, vitamin B17 found in apple, cherry, grape, peach, and apricot seeds, as well as Essiac tea, an herbal tonic comprised of burdock root, sheep sorrel, slippery elm, and turkey rhubarb, are looked at as just another attempt by the alternative health care community to undermine years of research from the most prestigious authorities in the world. EXACTLY!!!!

    Scientific research is lost in their own dogma. Why are the breast cancer rates in the United States five times higher than those in Japan? Would the elevated consumption of fish, rich in omega-3 essential fatty acids have anything to do with it? Why aren't Laetrile, Essiac Tea, and essential fatty acids being investigated with the same intensity and backing as Western, medical methods? Why were Doctor Dansbach, a pioneer in oxygen and nutritive therapies, and Doctor Hoxey, who used herbal formulas to treat cancer patients, forced to flee to Mexico to continue their work? Why were they persecuted and their methods systematically suppressed? What are our cancer institutions afraid of? Why won't they investigate every possibility available to them?

    This does not mean that science and medicine are unqualified to dispute other methods of treating disease as long as it is not focused on simply implementing monopolistic conformity. We must be watchful not to become prisoners chained to the

---

[3] Ibid

dungeons of science. Science and technology are in fact useful ways to attain knowledge. Medicine can and should examine gene therapy. They should experiment with cutting edge pharmaceuticals. However, by trusting that traditional science is the only source of truth to behold, we are limiting ourselves to only that which science knows. Just because science has not detected a certain phenomenon does not mean it cannot exist. It only means our technology cannot detect it. Certainly there were microwaves present in the atmosphere before we discovered a way to harness them and heat our food. Are we to believe that ultraviolet rays did not exist before man discovered them?

Medical science cannot explain the miracle of the evolving fetus yet the fetus develops anyway. How does, at conception, that one cell proliferate into a living human being? How does that growing mass of similar cells know when to differentiate? Who directs the development of the organs and how does your liver always wind up on the right side? How do the toe nails get to the tops of the toes? All this happens without the intervention of medicine, yet medicine wants us to believe that they and they alone hold the answers to life and well-being.

Why are we the only creature on earth that requires doctors to monitor our entire process of conception and delivery? Pregnancy is treated like a disease complete with medical intervention, without which would presumably leave us and our newborn baby both doomed.

Ultrasounds, fetal-monitoring, episiotomies, C-sections, amniocentesis, antibiotics, and immediate exposure to vaccines are just some of the tools used to intervene in what is a natural phenomenon to every other animal on earth.

Hospitals are standing by the ready to put silver nitrate into your newborn's eyes. Why? It is used to prevent the gonorrheal infection that the mother has from infecting the baby's eyes as the baby passes through the birth canal. What? Are the hospitals assuming that every mother has gonorrhea? Mom has been under a doctor's close supervision for nine months. Don't you think that if mom was infected that this would have been revealed on some test by now? These kinds of routine procedures assume that every single case needs a super hero to save us from destruction. Being the smartest creature on earth does not mean we have to intercede in the natural process of childbirth and turn it into pathology.

Do you realize that man is the only living entity that could become extinct today and not adversely affect the outcome of the planet? Every other living organism has a place in this web of life and obeys nature's laws. These organisms act in ways that are innately endowed to them. Giraffes do not need throat lozenges. Hyenas are not prescribed Ritalin. Rabbits do not require episiotomies. Monkeys do not feast on antibiotics when they catch colds. Elephants do not need antacids. Flowers bloom without growth hormones. Drastic changes in weather patterns do not need to be analyzed by a psychiatrist to be declared unstable. Life happens in spite of all our scientific research and man's endless tampering.

We, as humans, have the same innate ability to maintain ourselves in a state of health as any other animal. Our bodies respond to the same natural processes as do the aforementioned groups. We are a part of, not apart from, this world. We are bound to the interactions of yin and yang, give and take, life and death, up and down, alpha and omega, as every other living entity is. Experts are trapped in man-made laws and fear that breaking them may expose their own ineptitude. Those who operate under Natural Law have a deep trust in their own innate wisdom and understanding. It is the same guided wisdom that tells a seed that it needs to grow upward towards the sun. It is the same source that directs the deer to perk up its ears and flee when it senses danger.

The answers to life, in the medical-scientific model's perspective, all rest in reprogramming our genes, creating artificial immunity through vaccines, altering our food with biotechnology, surgically removing parts of our anatomy that are deemed dispensable, and labeling germs as harmful conduits of disease which then need to be completely eradicated. All of these are contrary to the circle of life and supporting natural phenomenon.

A television commercial espousing the benefits of aspirin on the cardiovascular system suggests, "Take it for pain, take it for life." There is no balance between all this scientific contemplation and a comprehension of innate intelligence. The medical minded fortress is attempting to convince us that the only thing that can save your heart is aspirin. This assumption is beyond ludicrous. They have completely disavowed the healing properties of Mother Nature's gifts in the form of vitamin E, calcium and magnesium, garlic, and Co-Q10. We need to look through the bias research studies, past the God complexes that pervade medicine, and beyond the toxic pharmaceuticals that cover up symptoms and create more problems with side effects. Then we can begin to appreciate how easy it is to walk within the enterprise of health.

This is the very allegory taught to us in the Garden of Eden. Adam and Eve inhabited a world of glorious perfection. The word Eden itself is used even today to describe a utopian environment. They lived within a world of complete faith and understanding of their quintessence. Life was not questioned. Life just existed perfectly as it was. The flawlessness of the world was shown to them through their own divinity. As soon as the tree of knowledge was partaken of, their world forever changed for the worse. That is to say, when Adam and Eve began to ask questions and look inquisitively into their own existence, they fell from grace. They traded in their intuition and faith based utopia for analysis, doubt, and a need for reason. By using this symbolism of the ancients we can come to better understand our own evolution of consciousness and recreate our world once again.

The interplay between yin and yang is replete in every facet of life. We inhale, we exhale. We sleep, we rise. Winter cools, summer warms. Yin and yang is the interplay of feminine and masculine, darkness and light, birth and death. It is seen in the rain that wets the earth and the evaporation that moistens the sky. There is a rhythmic cycle of give and take, up and down, in and out, that dictates the chorus of existence. This natural phenomenon was choreographing the planet's orbits and the patterns of the stars long before man invented Valium. Food chains existed and species adhered to them way before osteoporosis was created. By holding fast to some basic tenets of Natural Law and by applying some common sense to our lives, we can markedly improve our health status without the costly intervention of medical doctors and hospitals.

My system of health care is one that fuses to a living structure that has been in effect for eons of time. It relates to natural flow predicated on divine perfection. It incorporates the spirit into healing. Without it, there is no animation, no life.

My system of health care acknowledges emotions as real and viable form of pathological origin. I do not force upon my patients big, fancy, Latin rooted diagnoses. My system of health care talks in terms of energy and uses analogies to natural happenstance. I do not dissect my patients into parts. If we have gout, our big toe is not the only part of us that is sick. High cholesterol does not just affect our arteries. A kidney stone does not only represent a sick kidney. Every cell in our body is deprived of its perfection and senses the imbalance. This intrusion is detected everywhere and the condition becomes a concern to every cell that comprises our being.

"The cure for many diseases is unknown to the physician because they are ignorant of the whole...for the part can never be well unless the whole is well."

Plato

I have been chastised not only by medical professionals but also from within my own peer group for using words like spirit, energy, love, emotion, passion, and espousing Natural Law. But let me ask you some questions. How are those drugs working for you? Have they cured anything or merely extinguished some nagging symptoms. How long have you been on Imitrex for your migraines? How much longer will you tolerate them before you try another approach? Does your Lipitor control your cholesterol? What will happen if you stop taking it? Has it really cured anything? How's that methotrexate therapy coming along? Have you seen the warning in the *Physician's Desk Reference* for methotrexate? This is not your run of the mill list of side effects and contraindications. Did you ever wonder why your liver functions needed to be tested while on this drug? Does a fatal toxic reaction worry you? Deaths have been reported in the use of methotrexate in the treatment of psoriasis. Vitamin E and zinc are great tools to heal the skin and they have never killed anyone. Regardless of scientific naysayers, I have successfully treated all of these conditions (and more) with faith in Natural Law as prescribed through the tenets of chiropractic, acupuncture, aboriginal wisdom, electromagnetic technology, and whole food supplements. No drugs, no side effects, no problem!

When I was in high school, we would exchange gossip, talk about our soccer team's latest victory and trade information about the most recent test results during our breaks. Today our children swap their asthma inhalers with the same regularity and no one bats an eye. Children carrying inhalers are as common today as my generation was in carrying calculators to algebra class. Ritalin fills their pockets instead of spare change or a bag of M&M's. If this is the best that medical science can offer, count me out.

How much information have you heard of connecting ADD with nutritional deficiencies? In the 1940's, an eight ounce can of Pepsi contained two serving. Today, we are confronted with 64 ounce super sizes. In 2003 our annual consumption of sugar had morphed to an astronomical 142 pounds per person.[4] This overdosing of refined sugar and high fructose corn syrup has a profound effect on brain chemistry as well as sleep disturbance and immune system suppression. Can this have anything to do with the increasing rates of ADD? Medicine wants us to believe it doesn't. Just keep taking your drugs. Everything will be fine.

Why is something as simple as acid reflux labeled a disease? Acid reflux is not a disease. It is a condition of dis-ease. It is a body that is not at ease with its own routine digestive function. We have been told that it results from too much stomach acid which regurgitates up into the esophagus. What if I told you that acid reflux was the complete opposite, that is was due to not enough acid in the stomach. Without enough acid and enzymes in our stomach, the food we recently consumed sits in the stomach and rots. This rotting food, like the nearby landfill, emits toxic gas from the putrefying matter and upsets the whole community. If you accept the medical definition of acid reflux, then you accept the fact that as we age every function of our body slows down ***except*** the production of stomach acid. Stomach acid is the only factor that actually speeds up as we age? Acid reflux is a digestive system

---

[4] "One Sweet Nation." 3/28/05.
<http://www.usnews.com/usnews/health/articles/050328/28sugar.b.htm>

that is void of enzymes and a nervous system that is not stimulating the acid secretion of the stomach. It is poor food choices. It is entirely something we can control and cure. Antacids will not improve the digestive capacity of our stomach. They will only further diminish our stomachs ability to break down the food by decreasing an already depleted enzyme and acid repository. Medicine will only treat the symptom and never address the cause of the symptom itself.

Western medicine has also exonerated chronic fatigue and irritable bowel into the league of syndromes. Once labeled as a syndrome, the condition becomes more solidified in our consciousness. It takes on more importance. We are programmed to believe a cure is out of reach and medical intervention is the only option.

Fibromyalgia and Lupus, likewise, are not conditions in which you are enslaved unto for the rest of our life. They are manifestations of imbalances in our energetic program, stress imposed through the nervous system, and deficiencies in our dietary discrimination. They, too, will respond to the nurturing effects of the earth medicines as directed through chiropractic, acupuncture, whole foods, fresh water, and exercise.

I must question the medical Trojan horse's blatant disregard for other healing modalities. I see the hypocrisy in a profession that informs the public that if we go to a chiropractor once we will have to go back for the rest of our lives. They do not understand the foundation of chiropractic. One of chiropractic's many functions is in the capacity of preventative care; the exact same way we brush your teeth to avoid cavities and we change our motor oil to protect our car's engine from breakdown. Chiropractic adjustments can help prevent premature degeneration in our body the same way a front end alignment on our car prevents the tires from wearing improperly.

If the medical profession were to look in the mirror, they would see themselves creating the same co-dependent relationship with their own patients. The would begin by participating in the delivery of a baby, filling her with vaccines, performing well baby checkups, school physicals, mending a broken bone, testing for scoliosis, and prescribing Accuntane for acne. Seems pretty routine so far. However, Accutane can cause fetal defects in pregnant women so our teen age patient is put on birth control pills to prevent any mishaps. (Ever wonder what damage a medication does to *your* body when it is capable of causing fetal defects?) Then, because the side effects of Accuntane arise, depression and suicidal tendencies manifest. Our young lady is soon back in the doctor's office receiving a new prescription for Prozac. Another prescription is written to alleviate the new side effects from Prozac and the star of our story begins a vicious cycle of one side effect after another being covered up by one prescription after another.

      The accumulated toxic effects of the drugs eventually takes its toll and she soon finds herself riddled with chronic fatigue syndrome and fibromyalgia. It's back to the doctor's office who can only prescribe more drugs. In the midst of her own personal investigation, she learns of the relationship of fibromyalgia to gluten, dairy, and sugar. Unfortunately, her lifetime of dis-ease has allowed cancer to strike at the age of 55. By now, she has learned to explore other modalities of health and she comes across information concerning the relationship of birth control pills and increased incidence of certain cancers. In any event, sorry to say, her indoctrination into the medical world view has created too strong of a bond to overcome her fear and doubt of other therapies. The medical bias is ingrained into her psyche and she undergoes chemotherapy, radiation, and surgery. She dies seven years later. Believe me, once you go to an MD, *you will have to go back the rest of your life.* Where have I heard that before? Where is that eagle soaring above the mountain when you need it?

Doctors have routinely prescribed antibiotics to children with colds even though antibiotics do not kill viruses. Antibiotics only work on bacterial infections. In the early 1990's, because of the haphazard administration of antibiotics, we began to see the news media cover stories concerning super, drug resistant bacteria. This is another example of the limited vision of the scientific community. They found that a strain of bacteria could be eradicated by the administration of a particular form of drug therapy. Do not forget that bacteria are living, breathing life forms. They have a desire, as all living creatures do, to exist and propagate. They will find a way to survive. It is evolution at its best. The answer as to how to stop the super bacteria from proliferating does not lie in creating super antibiotics. You will only perpetuate the already serious problem.

What if we switched our focus from attacking and killing harmful bacteria to the promotion of helpful flora that resides in our bodies naturally? What if we built up our innate defenses to the point where harmful bacteria cannot take over? What if we stopped fighting natural processes and began working within the constructs of life's own divine paradigm? I have not been to see a medical doctor for over 20 years. I have faith in my circulatory system's ability to regulate my blood pressure every second of every day. I understand that my digestive system will change the food I eat into my own flesh and blood. I believe in my immune system and that it will be able to fight off an innocuous cold without a prescription. I know that with a nervous system clear of stress my body can adapt to changes and perform exactly in the manner in which it was designed.

I know that nutrition plays an indispensable role in our health. I know that oxygen is a necessity of life and the less pure it becomes, the less healthy you will be. I know our bodies are comprised mostly of water for a reason. That reason needs to be acknowledged and we must keep hydrated to keep healthy. I know the value of a nervous system that can understand changes in our internal and external environments and process the information without any interference. I believe that energetic frameworks surround our bodies and are as much a part of us as is our teeth, lungs and skin, regardless of whether our scientists have proven its existence. I do not required specialized instrumentation to emphatically prove inspiration or intuition. I adapt to the seasonal changes without complaint as do all other creatures. My body's innate intelligence controls my hormones and sugar levels without a prescription from the AMA. The physiological wisdom granted to me at conception flows from above-down, inside-out, as directed by forces that can never be genetically cloned or replaced by a synthetic pharmaceutical. I am part of the web of life and will never be a master of it.

Please do not misunderstand me when I speak adversely of the medical community. I am not admonishing the entire profession as misguided know-it-alls. Medicine has its place. Without question it has certainly saved lives. Our system of emergency care is state of the art. Our life saving, critical care is the best in the world. When you are in the throes of a heart attack or bleeding to death from a compound fracture of your femur, no herb and no chiropractic adjustment will stop the demise. Some conditions warrant medical mediation. Most do not.

It is sad in a way (and exactly my point) that I have to make the following disclaimer: I am in no way telling you that medical doctors are never to be utilized. Someone somewhere will read this book and ignore the pain in his lower right quadrant. He will rub some castor oil on it but to no avail. When his appendix burst and he dies of septicemia, I will be the first one his lawyer calls. This is where the very important dose of common sense and responsibility comes into play. Each one of us is 100% responsible for the choices we make. We cannot blame McDonalds because we are obese. We cannot blame the storefront owner because, in the middle of the winter, we slipped on some ice in front of their store.

It is common knowledge that winter freezes the elements and therefore we must be more aware of our surroundings. We cannot blame cigarette companies for our cancer nor the gun manufacturer for the accidental death of a family member. Our choices are just that. They are ours and ours alone. By making our choices wisely we will reap the rewards. There is a time and a place for medicine but it is not every time and everyplace. We are all too willing to blindly follow the medical community's recommendations without any form of contemplation.

It is becoming more apparent that when it comes to common sense, the people of this country, and the world for that matter, are becoming more and more deficient. I remember a commercial on television in which a gentleman is driving his RV and notices a sporty new car coming up from behind him. He leaves the driver's seat to race to the back of the RV and watch the sports car zoom past. Then he dashes back to his driver's seat before his wife wakes up to witness his actions. It is a silly commercial and I understood that the driver's actions were not to be taken seriously. Yet, the advertiser's needed to scroll a disclaimer across the screen stating, "Don't try this in your motor home." This only reinforced the diminished level of common sense we have sunk to.

My focus here is to point out that there are some simple things we can do to take care of ourselves first and foremost to ward off the coming of old age, illness, and the conditions associated with them. None of us want to spend our golden years wrapped up in a diaper or tethered to an oxygen tank. There isn't anyone out there who prays for the day to come when they can forgo the freedom of mobility for a walker. There are better choices for us and our health care and many of them have been kept from us by facades of politics and bias. What we know about conventional medicine and its relationship to health is only one side of the story. There are options available to us and it is up to us to use our personal freedom of choice to make an educated decision as to how we want to framework the quality of our life. There is no law that says you must suffer infectious disease or chronic, degenerative conditions. We can make free willed decisions as to how we will approach our health concerns.

We can reclaim our innate right to health by adhering to some simple measures of common sense. In the chapters to follow, I will talk to you in basic terms of understanding. I will not bury you in a morass of scientific analysis. I will not quote the latest research from the Mayo Clinic concerning some enzyme in the alpha stage of liver detoxification. I will, instead, expose you to some fundamental facts and relate them to the world around you. I will pose some basic questions that will make you rethink your position. I will revive the common sense approach to health. My words will resonate with that part of you that just knows the difference between right and wrong and creates discernment without having to be analyzed twelve different ways, biopsied for a diagnosis, and printed in a peer review journal.

"Natural forces are the healers of disease."
Hippocrates

CHAPTER FIVE

DID CURIOSITY KILL THE CAT OR MAKE HIM KING OF THE FOREST?

"I must create a system for myself, or be the slave of some other man's."
William Blake

All this questioning and this form of thinking have enabled me to see beyond the paradigm of the status quo. I do not believe that any one way to accomplish a task is the only way. The infinite brilliance that has come together to form life is not limited to one dimension, one definition. When working within life's never-ending grandeur, as a healer does, one cannot be successful if one's thinking becomes linear and does not mirror the original, boundless essence that creates all life.

In my youth, my tormented mind was a blessing in disguise. It allowed me the freedom to question. It gave me a sense of open-mindedness that few can appreciate. It permitted me to see the world in a different regard. With the application of our sight, smell, taste, touch, and hearing and the molding from our culture, we have defined our space in the world. But I came to understand that our human perception is not the only way to define reality. What if we could speak to the animals? What if we asked one of the bats that lived in our barn to define its world? The bat would describe its existence as a system or a series of sonar blips and beeps. A bumblebee from my mother's flower garden would show us a world that vibrates and pulses in ultraviolet lights. So what is reality and who defines it? Even we humans have different definitions of reality.

Ask 100 people to describe the perfect vacation and you will get 100 different answers. No two people experience the same reality.

I was approaching my teen years when I first began to contemplate a world beyond what our limited senses could detect. I began to see a world that my inquisitive mind could comfortably fit into. My stepfather had back surgery in 1977 to repair some bulging discs in his lumbar spine. As part of his rehabilitation, he was introduced to the world of bio-energetics. He learned about biofeedback methods to control pain. He learned about the energetic systems of the body and how to manipulate those energies. He brought these gifts home with him as well as knowledge about meditative relaxation techniques and a powerful skill in massage. I found this concept of healing intriguing to say the least. It fueled my already questioning mind and lead me on a journey like no other. It taught me to look beyond the tangible world and begin to appreciate the intangible, invisible, energetic, animating life forces.

Do you remember those pictures that became popular in the 1990s that appeared to be just a psychedelic collage of mixing, swirling colors? We had to train our eyes to look through the colors to see the three-dimensional picture hidden within it. With this slight change of focus, a world within a world is exposed to the viewer. This is a great tool to use to explain how to appreciate the energetic world that exists within our visible, physical world. With a slight shift in our senses, we can realize an existence in another dimension. This energy work that my stepfather introduced me to, proved to me that there was indeed a world beyond our limited perception, one that was full of infinite possibilities. It was one with no manmade boundaries or expectations.

These events taught me that there is no one answer to my questions. Whether religious, historical, political, and especially medical, there are infinite possibilities available to us. If God, the source of all life, is omnipresent, omnipotent, and omniscient, how can people confined health and healing to only one limited technique? Health, healing, and life are as boundless as the source that created it. Understanding that lies in how we fine-tune and apply our senses. It lies in our willingness to be open-minded and receive this information. It is about having a heart that resonates with the truth, with the Big Picture.

As a wellness consultant, acupuncturist, and chiropractor, I have been exposed to numerous pathologies over my professional career. I have treated patients with musculoskeletal disorders, chemical imbalances, nutritional deficiencies, emotional issues, and organic dysfunction. The vast majority of my patients have come to me as a last resort. I hear patient after patient relive their medical history with a desperate voice and a hopeful heart. Most have already been diagnosed by a medical doctor and treated without success. They have been poked and prodded and examined with all the latest technology that insurance companies will pay for. Most have gone through round after round of pharmaceuticals with the words "If this doesn't help, come back and see me in two weeks" ringing in their ears. Others have been given the obligatory "You are getting old and you will just have to learn to live with it," or "There is nothing more that can be done." I have witnessed first-hand this medical mismanagement propagated through the ignorance of the ego and the blindness of medical-political tradition.

Why is that? Our medical system is focused on there being a physical cause for a physical problem. If our condition cannot be physically analyzed then modern medicine is at a loss. When all the tests come back and our blood work is normal, our x-rays are negative, and our physical exam is unremarkable, medicine has nothing more to offer. This is because our existence is comprised of more than just a physical body.

What about our emotional body? We love our pet dog or cat but love cannot be proven by science. Does that mean our emotions have no bearing on our health? What about our energetic body? Have we ever walked into a crowded room and were immediately drawn to one particular person? How does this energetic phenomenon relate to our being or to our health? Your spiritual body has influence upon us as well. What motivated us to give up our Thanksgiving celebration to work in a soup kitchen for the day? Did our spiritual body create the thought that told us to donate time to our community and pick up trash along the roadside? The emotional, energetic, and spiritual parts of our existence are just as real as our physical parts. They influence our life just as much as the sunshine warms our body in the summer time. Medicine, however, disavows any role that these types of bioenergetics may play in establishing health. Why? What is medicine trying to hide? What are they afraid of?

"Our Deepest fear is not that we are inadequate. Our deepest fear is that we are powerful beyond measure. It is our light, not our darkness that most frightens us."
Marianne Williamson

The disastrous state of our health care system stems in part from the establishment's continual desire to look into the body for that one magic bullet that has caused the entire problem. The medical model separates us into pieces and dissects those pieces further and further until we have become nothing more than a single cell under a microscope. Medicine will have much more success if it turns its focus completely around and begins to examine not how each piece works by itself but rather how the human body acts as a whole. Medical research has spent so much time studying the microcosm, the tiniest, remotest frontiers of DNA, a bacterium, or virus that they have forgotten about our relationship to the macrocosm, to the world around us. They have tried in vain to discover the answers to life by separating our bodies into individual units: lungs, spinal cord, skin, and blood, forgetting that these individual units are exactly what have come *together* to evolve into this entity we call the human body. We are not the lower lobe of a lung. We are not nervous tissue. We are not flakes of skin and we are not a pool of blood. All of these elements unite as one to create our life. Health, healing, and life must include an understanding of the whole, the macrocosm, and the physical body's relationship to itself as well as the energetic world if it wishes to perpetuate.

As we cannot separate the parts of our body and expect them to act as sole proprietor, neither can we separate the human condition from the rest of existence. As all our cells have bound together to create our body, our body then becomes a cell in the body of life. As our red blood cells traverse our vascular system interacting with all the other tissues, we as whole human beings must traverse life interacting with all the other life forms. The tiniest forms of life have the same interactions as the largest forms of life. Understanding how humans react and respond to life outside themselves will help them understand how their cells respond and react within themselves.

Our existence is composed of a physical, chemical, emotional, energetic, and spiritual nature. Though we can describe these different layers of our existence as single entities, ultimately these layers all originates from the same source. If we can tap into that original source we can better understand the processes of life itself. The source of life is not bound up in a green pill nor is it awash in cough syrup. The source of life cannot be dissected from the body or cultured in a state-of-the-art laboratory.

To begin to understand the energetic realm of life, we can look to nature to get a glimpse of this spirit in action. Then, like the aforementioned pictures of the swirling colors, change our perception a bit and look through the physical qualities of nature and sense the energetic world within the physical world. By doing so, the activities of the physical world soon become rhythmic and we can begin to sense patterns. We are not literally using our superpower x-ray vision to physically look through a tree. Rather, we are attempting to tap into the ebb and flow of nature's inherent, perfect expression of itself. These patterns can help to foster energetic intuition. That is the perceptive insight that allows a healer to heal through analogy. The energetic patterns in nature that sustain life are the same energetic patterns in our bodies. The microcosm is the macrocosm.

As I discussed earlier, looking at the world differently is not a new phenomenon. Paradigms have changed numerous times over the course of history. Isaac Newton, Albert Einstein, Jesus Christ, and Thomas Jefferson all created new paradigms with their new forms of thought. At one time, our science and religion centered on the assumption that the earth was the center of the solar system. Copernicus proved that assumption wrong. Medical science once believed that mercury was a curative. Now we know it is a toxic heavy metal that can cause brain damage. These are but a few examples of changes in thinking that have altered our outlook of the planet.

Our health care system will not improve until we awaken our senses and change our perceptions of it. We must take back the control of our own health and become responsible for our actions. We must make choices that promote life, love, and happiness and shun those choices that do not. We must no longer allow the AMA to monopolize the health care industry and exclude other forms of healing (of which they have been found guilty of in a court of law three separate times: first in 1937 for trying to destroy the newly forming health insurance idea, secondly in 1982 for systematic violation of antitrust statutes, and thirdly in 1987 for conspiring to destroy and eliminate the chiropractic profession.)

Medicine must accept quantum physics and the electromagnetic properties of our existence as a valid basis for life. Medicine must no longer look at life through a reductionist's microscope, dissecting parts into smaller pieces, and isolating one gene against another. Medicine must shift its work to include holism and appreciate the interconnectedness of life in its multitude of expressions.

"When in the course of human events it becomes necessary for one people to dissolve the political bands which have connected them with another and to assume among the Powers of the earth, the separate and equal station to which the **Laws of Nature** *and of* **Nature's God** *entitle them, a decent respect to the opinions of mankind require that they should declare the cause which impel them to separation."*
The Declaration of Independence

When I work with patients, I use energetics as an intricate part of my diagnosing and treating. When I speak of energy, I am using it as a synonym for frequency or vibration. The atomic vibrational frequency of a substance determines its density and its functional expression as matter. This is the only difference between ice, water, and steam. They are all molecularly identical. Only the speed at which their molecules vibrate is different. Ice has a low vibrational essence and a greater density. Water has a higher vibrational essence (it moves more freely) and is less dense. The molecules of steam have the greatest vibration of the three, and steam is even less dense than the water. The faster molecules vibrate the less physical they become. Our bodies act in the same manner as the ice. A dead body has no vibrational essence and is most dense, like ice. While we are alive we can be compared to the water. We are moving and fluid. Our souls, angels, ghosts or any description of the afterlife are akin to the steam. Both the steam and our souls have an intangible quality, a nonphysical form, an ethereal appearance to them. Though the steam, as well as our own souls, appears to be more energy-based and less physical, a simple change in the speed at which the molecules vibrate will expose a different form of the same character.

There is more to diagnosis than just observing how the symbolic form of water runs. A healer must be able to see the patient as ice, water, and steam. Each layer of the patient can expose critical information needed in creating a treatment program. Maybe even more important than taking vital signs and listening to the patient's case history are the nonphysical elements involved in their expression. The action of the "steam" can be just as revealing. I see patients react to certain words. Their posture tells a story as do their own communication skills. Are they approachable or reserved? Are they stoic or emotional? I hear the inflections in their voices describe particular events. One can develop the skill not only to look through the physical condition and tap into the underlying energetic blueprint, but also to listen beyond the spoken words a patient uses and hear the tones that carry the words. I have seen a connection between a specific condition and its related emotional issue. As I was palpating a sore spot on a patient's neck she told me, "That feels familiar." She may have said *familiar* but I sensed the word *family*. This clued me in to ask questions pertaining to her parents. This, in turn, opened up a can of worms that inevitably helped her to resolve some emotional issues and the physical problems associated with them.

I have learned that nothing is as it seems on the outside. The physical representation of this world is a camouflage for a deeper, more energetic and mysterious, spiritual existence. Our body is a world within a world. Nature exhibits patterns in every aspect of its evolution. So do humans inasmuch we are just as much a part of nature as the tulips and grasshoppers. Poor health and illness can be directly linked to destructive patterns within natural, God-directed, purpose-driven, constructive patterns inherent in all life forms.

Because I can work within the world of nature's patterns, because I appreciate the give and take of life's processes, because I interpret physical language into metaphor, I can confidently predict which healing crisis may take place first on a patient's path to recovery. I can tell the patient what to expect and, sure enough, when they return for their follow up visit, they tell me, "You know, you were right."

Any medical establishment that wishes to discredit new age medicine, alternative medicine, energy work, or the spirituality of healing is just as eagerly trying to convince you that I do not exist. I have experienced all of these constituents in relationship to healing and can vow that they are as real as the smiles on our faces. If we choose not to accept the viability of natural medicine or the reality of energetic healing then we can continue to wash away symptom after symptom with a fog of medication. That is absolutely our choice. Those who denounce alternative medicine are fearful. They are afraid that the truth in healing will somehow discredit their own existence. What would happen to the integrity of the medical profession if they, right now, proclaimed that vaccinating every child for every disease may not be the best answer? They are afraid they will lose our trust and therefore our business.

"Perfect obedience to the laws of health would abolish the medical profession."
Octavius Brooks Frothingham

I have seen one chiropractic treatment reduce the muscles in a man's back from contracting severely in spasm every few minutes to only one spasm the entire next day. I have witnessed the power of acupuncture to restore a woman's capability to reproduce. I have prescribed proper whole food supplements to help cure psoriasis. I have seen the healing powers of an Ojibwa sweat lodge dissolve feelings of shame that a psychiatrist could not touch. These incidents occurred, of course, after all these people had been told by their respective doctors that there was nothing more that could be done for them. When a medical doctor tells you that the only choice for your carpal tunnel syndrome is surgery, they are wrong. When you are told by the Mayo Clinic that there is no cure for Meniere's disease, you have been given a prognosis through bias eyes. When pediatricians state your baby will outgrow the colic, they are not in tune with the Big Picture.

    This healing paradigm I speak of lies within the very source of life itself. It is the understanding of the Big Picture. You may be wondering how I define this source of life, this Big Picture I elude to. It is the humble concession to a greater creative power and a belief that this phenomenon has infinitely more wisdom concerning the processes of life than man will ever, ever comprehend.

    Understanding the Big Picture is knowing that the intricacies of the process of life are infinitely more than man's finite thinking can comprehend. This truth comes to us when we respectfully and gratefully accept our pre-ordained perfection, realize our potential, and allow that realization to manifest our purpose. This truth is embedded in the natural process of life and death. Life and death, alpha and omega, yin and yang, all originate from the source of creation and all creation dances to the song of the spirit. Life goes on with or without man. It existed before man and will continue to flourish when man is gone. Truth knows that there is a power fused within all life that can be expressed in more than just physical terms. It is accepting that spirit is in control of all life's processes. That is the Big Picture. We can hop on board and enjoy the ride or we can live our life in a quagmire of fear and doubt. Nature is the master of man, not the other way around.

Bartlett Joshua Palmer, the most powerful and influential of all chiropractors, defined truth in relation to the chiropractic paradigm in this manner:

> *We chiropractors work with the subtle substance of the soul. We release the imprisoned impulse, the tiny rivulet of force that emanates from the mind and flows over the nerves to the cells and stirs them to life. We deal with the majestic power that transforms common food into living, loving, thinking clay that robes the earth with beauty and hues and scents the flowers with the glory of the air.*
>
> *In the dim, dark, distant, long ago, when the sun first bowed to the morning star, this power spoke and there was life. It quickened the slime of the sea and the dust of the earth and drove the cell to union with its fellows in countless living forms. Through eons of time it finned the fish and winged the bird and fanged the beast. Endlessly it worked, evolving its form until it produced the crowning glory of them all. With tireless energy it blows the bubbles of each individual life and then silently, relentlessly, dissolves the form and absorbs the spirit into itself again.*
>
> *And yet you ask, "Can chiropractic cure appendicitis or the flu? Have you more faith in a spoonful of medicine than in the power that animates the living world?"*

It is from this mindset that I relate how our health is a direct reflection of the capacity to understand and work within the constructs of the natural rhythms and cycles of the world. It is from here that I explain the spirituality of breathing, the necessity of eating real, whole foods, and the importance of energetic body work. I will emphasize the importance of oxygen and the fact that sitting on the couch six hours a day does nothing to infuse the body's tissues with this gaseous gold. I hope to create an attitude that will not accept the irrational thinking of food manipulators- that the stripping of our food of its innate perfection through processing, adding toxic bleach, and fortifying it with synthetic pseudo-vitamins has everything to do with disease and nothing to do with health. My goal is to show how a physical body becomes a manifestation of an energetic blueprint, and these energies can be redefined to promote longevity, happiness, and health.

My perspective on health is simpler than the perspective suggested by the Western medical model. It is based on my experience with the Ojibwa Indians of Northern Wisconsin, my studies of the art, science, and philosophy of chiropractic health care, and the teachings of traditional Chinese medicine. These three entities are firmly rooted in Natural Law. They adhere to tenets grounded in spirituality. They work within the confines of the process of life without trying to recreate what Mother Nature has already created. Does this make me an expert in natural healing? No, not even close. What it does make me is someone who understands the processes that build life and knows that every living cell on earth obeys them without question. An oak tree in Minnesota does not rebel and keep its leaves green all winter. A caterpillar does not decide to change into a frog while wrapped up in its cocoon. Nature allows its infinite forms to manifest effortlessly. I know that humans are part of this magical dance called life not separate from it or master of it. We, therefore, are regulated under the same divine plan as every bumble bee, sperm whale, magpie, pumpkin, and blade of grass. We are so connected to nature that a healthy woman's menstrual cycles is in direct synchronicity with the phases of the moon. Aboriginal women have "moon time" not periods.

This country's health care system is out of control. Many elderly cannot afford prescription drugs. We need to establish a level of accountability in regard to the profit made by pharmaceutical companies. We need to question why it costs drug companies about two-and-a half cents to make 100 Xanax when the sale price for the same amount hovers at $136.00. Millions of Americans cannot afford basic health insurance coverage. A trip to the emergency room can easily cost $1,000 or more. The miracle and joy of delivering a baby can run couples into debt to the tune of tens of thousands of dollars. People are developing degenerative illness at younger and younger ages. Something is definitely wrong with this picture.

If we keep ignoring this madness, we will further destroy the quality of our lives. There is no system of checks and balances. Doctors charge exorbitant fees. Insurance companies limit which modality of healing will be reimbursed and by how much. This country does not need socialized medicine to cure its ills. Dumping more tax money into our health care system will only reinforce an already deteriorating infrastructure. What we need is freedom of health care to accompany our other freedoms granted in the Constitution. What we need is a new paradigm, a new outlook on health, and this book will outline just what is required to free us from the stranglehold of the ogres called conventional medicine and managed health care.

"The Constitution of this Republic should make provisions for healing freedom as well as religious freedom. To restrict the art of healing to one class of men and deny equal privileges on others will constitute the Bastille of medical science. Such restrictions are fragments of monarchy and have no place in a Republic."
Benjamin Rush

CHAPTER SIX

A DIPLOMA DOES NOT A DOCTOR MAKE

"Familiar as the voice of the mind is to each, the highest merit we ascribe to Moses, Plato, and Milton is that they set at naught books and tradition, and spoke not what men, but what they thought. The writer, who takes his subjects from his ear and not from his heart, should know that he has lost as much as he has gained."
Ralph Waldo Emerson

The word doctor does not mean "I went to school forever and therefore I know everything." The root word translates from Latin and means teacher. The ancient doctors would teach their patients about living in harmony and in balance with nature. They taught people how healthy lifestyle choices could cure their ills. They did not demand adherence to self-imposed protocol. Organized medicine has now become an elite group of individuals demanding that we all must kowtow to their dictates. Today's organized medicine is a far cry from its original role as teacher. I, however, do not believe medical doctors merit any more importance than do librarians, fire fighters, or trash collectors. I lived in Philadelphia in 1986 when the garbage collectors went on strike for three weeks. Believe me; trash collection is just as important as any other job.

There are great doctors and there are lousy doctors. Some doctor's intentions are noble and others are driven by greed. Medicine has contributed much to our lives but it is also steeped in failures. Their profession is no different than the one you or I are currently enrolled in. Doctors are people just like you and I and therefore are endowed with the God given right to err. They are not perfect and they do not know all there is to know about health. Being a medical doctor does not give them the right to monopolize the health care industry by creating laws that perpetuate their own agenda. It does not give them the right to declare what is "scientific" and therefore deemed valid, nor does it give them the right to declare, via insurance claims, what is "medically necessary."

I always find it interesting when an examining board for an insurance company denies a chiropractic claim due to the claim not being a "medical necessity" without ever examining the patient's case file. In any event, chiropractors do not practice "medicine" and therefore nothing we do is a "medical necessity." The situation can be, however, a "chiropractic necessity!" Medical doctors will never comprehend this difference because they do not understand, nor do they want to understand, the chiropractic philosophy. Chiropractic philosophy is based on Natural Law not man made law and therefore it is deemed not scientific.

Doctors are granted diplomas on their ability to pass tests and demonstrate competency in certain fields. That does not grant them a degree in bedside manner. A passing test score does not fill them with a specific level of compassion. Wisdom is not disseminated at graduation. Twelve years of schooling does not guarantee any sense of inner awareness. It means you have read a lot of books and passed a lot of tests. Inner awareness does not come from dogma entrenched in tradition and bound in a text. It comes by understanding man's place in the Big Picture and applying that understanding in accordance with all other life through Natural Law. Wisdom comes to us through our senses and is transformed into experience. It is not a framed diploma hanging on a wall. Inner awareness is a vision of perfection which lies behind an imperfect sense of reality. You can begin to tap into this awareness, not by taking tests, but when you begin to focus on what makes us live rather than what makes us die. This sense, this awareness, is an attunement with the essence that creates and directs all forms of life.

> *"The only true wisdom is knowing you know nothing."*
> Socrates

What does all this talk of energy really mean? What's wrong with just existing in a physical world without quantum physics clouding up our comfort zone? Without the addition of quantum physics, the energetics of life, the complete understanding of health and life will never be ours to own. Let me try and bring all this talk of vibrational frequencies or essence into an understandable form that we can use.

There is an experiment we did in high school physics class in which we would drop two identical marbles from the same height, at the same time, into a container of water. We would then examine the waves thus created. Waves are a visible form of vibrations or frequencies. When the two separate waves meet, they combine into one larger wave. They resonated with each other creating greater amplitude.

By understanding the role of quantum physics and vibrational frequencies within the Big Picture, within nature, your own existence can resonate with those already established frequencies of life and create greater amplitude. Simply put, living in accordance with nature's laws, instead of man's laws, adds to your own sense of energy or vibrational essence. The combination of matching frequencies resonating within the constructs of life compliments and strengthens each other. Apples, fresh water, clean air, the application of chiropractic care, and other natural healing arts resonate with life and love. They all originate from the same creative life force, that being nature, and therefore they amplify each other's frequencies. As a healer, the "medicine" becomes stronger because it works in concert with that power from which life springs from originally.

On the other hand, by changing any one of the parameters of the experiment (size of the marble, height, timing), you will create two waves of varying frequencies. When these waves meet they cancel each other out. Their amplitude diminishes. That is to say, if your perception of life does not match the frequencies that support life, your "medicine" will weaken. Synthetic vitamins, man-made pharmaceuticals, cigarettes, pesticides, food additives, air pollution, and toxic water do not resonate with life. They are contaminated with man's intervention. They are not born from a natural source and therefore their frequencies do not match life enhancing energies. Hence they create chaos. The combined amplitude is diminished. This decrease in energy does not complement each other and leads to death.

Another way to explain matching frequencies is with the piano. Of the 88 keys presented, let's say that some of the keys represent whole foods, clean water, fresh air, exercise, holistic medicine, and all things natural. The others keys represents MSG, pharmaceuticals, benzene, aspartame, synthetic vitamins, artificial hormones, and all things man made. By combining notes within the natural keys, all tones complement each other and the music resonates with a luxurious, harmonic quality. Be careful. If you strike the wrong key, one of the man-made keys, the notes becomes sour. It does not resonate with the rest of the music. Its vibrational quality takes away from the perfection of the music.

Medical doctors cannot accept that I was responsible for helping Mona recover from severe, chronic psoriasis when their attempts had all failed. They cannot accept that I helped Barbara's anxiety attacks become so rare that she began socializing again when traditional methods had proven helpless.
Jill's migraines are gone after suffering through ten years of failed drug intervention. Kathy's fibromyalgia is

no longer just "under control" with drugs. She is totally "in control" of her life. When chiropractic helps to cure chronic endometriosis or acupuncture allows an asthmatic to breathe freely without medicine, a shock is delivered to the scientific community. They are bewildered to find that life does not behave as neatly as the laboratory model or the postmortem cadaver. The simple reason that medical doctors can not accept these anecdotes is because their experience has told them that it is impossible. The power of indoctrination has been imprinted on their psyche. Their current thought process does not allow them to see it. Even when they do physically see positive results from alternative therapies, their minds are not programmed to believe it.

"For you the world is weird because if you're bored with it, you are at odds with it. For me, the world is weird because it is stupendous, awesome, mysterious, unfathomable."
Don Juan in *Journey to Ixtlan* by Carlos Castaneda

Organized medicine (much like world religions) has separated itself from the cohesive bonds of conscious evolution. It remains content on only focusing on the differences within the multifaceted healing arts when in reality there is so much more in common. When we strip away the technical, specialized facade of today's medicine, we find that it is the same shamanistic practices of centuries ago. Only now it is defined in modern language and current technology. Modern medicine developed in the same manner as all other cultural healing techniques. It derived from people collecting experiences and using them to form patterns and explanation. These patterns serve to indoctrinate the healers into that particular form of healing. Whether a chiropractor, an internist, an acupuncturist, or a Reiki master, these experiences form a basis for interpretation. Interpretation can never be limited to only one mind set.

We all live in the same world but it is seen through different eyes and with different interpretation. Today, science has blended eons of cultural medicine into a brand of industrialized "one size fits all" medicine. But all new medicine must arise from prior archetypes. Are these archetypes really differentiated by linear years or are they the same aspects within parallel designs? Has evolution made modern medicine better or is it just a different application of the same old thing? As different as cultures are with their own traditions, languages, mythologies, rituals, foods, and tools, they all have a common thread that binds them together. It is the quest for understanding how the spirit transforms into matter or what the difference between life and death is. It is the desire to comprehend what forces animate life. Healing is based in the perennial questions; why are we here? Where did we come from? Where are we going? What makes us tick? Because of this basic concept that binds all of healing, healing cannot be generalized into a form of social casting and handed out through mass media. The answers to these questions can only be catalyzed (or impeded) by a medium, an interpreter. A healer translates these mystical questions into modalities that reflect the answers.

Organized medicine has gotten itself lost in the translation. They have separated themselves from the essence of these questions, from the essence of life and the powers that dictate its every move. When the patient's subjective complaints are still intact after medical intervention, where is the healing? For all those people who have been told that there is "nothing wrong with you," why do you still hurt? Maybe medicine has been looking in the wrong places for the answers to those age old questions mentioned above. Maybe the answers to health are not hidden in a cell wall of a bacterium. Maybe DNA is not the factor of predisposing us to disease. Maybe the homeostatic existence of one's life comes from an imbalance of a different nature (pun intended). Maybe by stripping away any semblance of a relationship to life's inherent interconnectedness, organized medicine has alienated itself from the very power that enables life to move forward. Maybe, just maybe. Medicine has been wrong before.

This disconnect that has manifest within organized medicine is replete and can be further exposed if one knows how to read between the lines. A brochure from the American Cancer Society states, "The best defense is to find breast cancer as early as possible when it is easiest to treat." Think about that statement. Is the best defense really to sit back and wait until breast cancer shows up? That's not a defense at all. Isn't the best defense against breast cancer to ward it off before it strikes? Wouldn't a more empowering statement such as, "There are numerous chemicals found in fresh fruits and vegetables that have been shown to keep cancer at bay," make more sense than waiting for the cancer to rear its devastating head? Where are the brochures from these cancer groups that proclaim the health benefits of exercise? Where is the proclamation that cancer cells are anaerobic and will die if exposed to oxygen? Waiting for the cancer to strike before we take action is a reactive response, not a defensive one, and certainly not a proactive one. These kinds of statements can only emphasize the erroneous thinking that permeates organized medicine.

Here's another example. An article published in the Wall Street Journal asserted that people who respond to the placebo effect are ruining clinical trials for drug companies. Drug companies want to exclude those participants from drug trials who respond favorably to the fake treatment or the sugar pill. It seems too many people are getting better only because they *think* they are getting treated. Here, organized medicine has a tremendous opportunity to research this incredible phenomena known as the placebo effect but instead chooses to completely ignore the power of the mind. Of course we can all see that this reaction from the drug companies is motivated by money. If we could teach our minds to heal disease we wouldn't need to spend billions of dollars on pharmaceuticals. Medicine would rather continue to promote the practice of introducing man-made chemicals into natural systems and pretend that the two are compatible.

I believe that for true healing to take place, the healer (whether the patient himself or someone assisting) must find that place where the body can once again reunite with the frequencies that sustain all of life. This kind of rhetoric is easy for us natural healers to toss around but what does it mean and how can the common folk apply it to everyday use? How does one reconnect with the vibrational frequencies of life? In the following chapters I will discuss these very issues and show you where health comes from and how easy it is to maintain. I will free you from the shackles of fear based propaganda directed through the medical industry.

"What hope is there for medical science to ever become a true science when the entire structure of medical knowledge is built around the idea that there is an entity called disease which can be expelled when the right drug is found?"
John H. Tilden

CHAPTER SEVEN

THE SEED VERSUS THE SOIL

"Nature is mythical and mystical always and works with the license and extravagance of genius."
Henry David Thoreau

If we are going to disregard the policy of ingesting toxic pharmaceuticals into our bodies merely to mask the signs and symptoms of dysfunction, what are our alternatives? If we accept the fact that God gave us all tonsils, an appendix, a gall bladder, and women a uterus for a reason, what else can we do when these "dispensable" organs fail to work properly? How do we stand up to infectious disease if we do not kill bacteria with every step we take? Should we have faith in natural immunity or should we create vaccines for every virus we discover? If medicine isn't our savior, how have we survived the onslaught of the new syndromes and complexes that emerge every year?

Part of the medical paradigm of health is rooted in seeking out and destroying germs. Medical science is in a constant attack mode always looking for that one agent, that one germ that may cause trouble. We must kill it before it kills us. In fact, through our patriarchal societies, this violent symbolism of aggression has permeated our entire culture. When you turn on the news, the headline story is, "Another attack in Iraq today kills three soldiers." Is fighting the enemy the only story to report in Iraq? Medicine, along with these news stories, does not focus on building a more stable foundation. They focus on the attacks, the war, the battle between good and evil. It is a testosterone driven model. What if we changed this attack mode thought process from fighting germs (or the enemy) to building health (or infrastructure?) What if we started to create desirable conditions that promote health and life rather than destroy undesirable conditions that are based in misunderstanding and fear? What if we started balancing all the testosterone based aggression with some estrogen based nurturing? Remember, balance is what makes nature perfect. As our thoughts change from attack to support, we will begin to see more stories like, "Garlic can help reverse heart disease," and "The women of Iraq are now going to school." As our thoughts change so will our world view, as I discussed earlier.

The medical establishment's propaganda machine has convinced us that antibiotics and vaccines are (note the common references to war here) the first line of defense in combating unwanted infectious germs. This fear of germs has snowballed into a state of overt ridiculousness. A commercial on television suggests that if we are using a dirty sponge we may as well be wiping off our counter tops with raw chicken, as the dirty sponge is loaded with germ spreading bacteria. If this scare tactic had any merit, we would have seen epidemics of "dirty sponge disease" years ago as generations of Americans have been utilizing dirty sponges for decades without any complications. Those same dirty sponge germs that we were all exposed to years and years ago as children are now deemed hazardous and we must take the necessary steps to avoid them.

A commercial on the radio endorses an antibacterial hand sanitizer. The ad tells us that every time we use the ATM we expose ourselves to a handful of cold hard E. Coli. Is it really such a necessity to carry hand sanitizer with us to the ATM? ATM's were introduced in the 1970's. With over 30 years of use without sanitizing our hands, where are the E. Coli epidemics? Can you see the fear based propaganda at play here?

More recently a television commercial showed two young girls wiping their pet dog with ordinary paper towels. One of the young girls then wipes the dog with a specially treated moist towel and shows the audience all the dirt that was picked up after the initial dry towel wiping. The sponsor then tries to sell us on the idea that "dry wiping" may not be enough to thoroughly clean ourselves. The people of this planet have been exclusively dry wiping themselves for centuries without any kind of "poor wiping" epidemics. Is this really a germ problem or is it a marketing ploy using fear based tactics?

The only epidemic here is one that I call germophobia; being afraid of innocuous germs. Here is yet another example. What is this obsession with having to wash your hands after you urinate? Try leaving a public restroom without washing your hands and the first emotion that pops into the back of your head is guilt. Others will stare in dismay as you disregard all sense of hygiene. Why? We have been conditioned to believe that not washing our hands after urinating is dirty. We have been brainwashed into believing that germs come from our bathroom habits and spreading these germs can cause disease. We become no better than a nasty infectious rat should we not wash our hands after urinating.

Let us now apply some logic to this scenario. We take a shower in the morning cleaning all our parts thoroughly, dry off with a clean towel, and slip on a pair of clean underwear. Everything under our clean underwear is now as germ free as it will be all day. The only time in which that part of our body greets the day for the rest of your waking hours is when we need to use the restroom. (Unless, of course, we are in a profession that warrants us to remove our clothing.) What germs are we afraid of here?

And if our hand should accidentally come into contact with a drop of urine, what's the problem? Urine is sterile. The thing of it is, our hands have been exposed to germs all day long. We have picked up the telephone, sneezed or coughed into our hands, and passed money through our fingers. We have shaken people's hands, touched doorknobs and handrails, and scratched our butt. Our hands are loaded with germs. When we go to the restroom, we should wash our hands first as to not spread germs from our filthy hands to our very clean private parts excreting sterile urine.

The medical establishment has constructed the Germ Theory of Disease based on previous work done by Louis Pasteur (from whom we pasteurize milk to kill germs), Joseph Lister (from whom we get the name Listerine which kills germs that cause bad breath), Edward Jenner (who created vaccines to kill germs), and Alexander Fleming (who discovered penicillin which kills germs). Wow! That's a lot of germ killing. I am surprised there are any germs left to kill. This Germ Theory of Disease blames germs for infectious disease. It states that:

1. The germ must be present in every case of the disease.
2. The germ must not be present in any other disease as an agent not responsible for that disease.
3. The germ must be capable of being isolated.
4. After growth in a pure culture, the germ must be able to reproduce the disease.

Basically, what the medical community wants us to believe is that, for example, the streptococcus bacillus causes strep throat every time, all the time, nothing else can cause strep throat, and if given the chance it will replicate and cause the same disease in someone else. This sounds familiar doesn't it? It is the story of spreading germs. Remember, this little postulate is the foundation of the medical profession. Let's examine it and see if it holds merit.

"If the germ theory of disease were correct, there would be no one left living to believe it."
B. J. Palmer

Yes, Doctor Palmer, how true. If germ "A" causes disease "A", every time, all the time, and is reproducible and transmittable, then we would all be dead from the Bubonic Plague.

Beginning in China in 1330 and spreading throughout the world via trade routes, Yersinia Pestis, the germ associated with Bubonic Plague, killed 1/3 of Europe's population. What happened to the other 2/3 of the population of Europe? Why didn't they "catch" the disease and die too? Were they all hiding in caves? Did they all move to Switzerland and remain neutral? How about the influenza epidemic of 1918? It killed 25 million people in one year. That's a very powerful little germ. Why weren't the rest of the planet's people infected?

The germ theory states that the germs can be isolated, replicated, and recreate the same disease. How did the survivors escape the wrath of these little monsters? There is a factor here that medicine did not include in their equation. That factor has to do with the vitality of the host organism. Spread all the germs you want, but if the host organism is healthy, the germ will be rendered insignificant by the host's immune system and not cause any harm. This includes germs as powerful as Yersinia Pestis and influenza.

We do not have to be forced to confide in an outdated theory. We can learn, expand our consciousness, and even change our way of thinking in regards to health and germs. Germs are not evil agents of infection blowing in the wind searching for a weakened prey. Bacteria are byproducts of dead and decaying tissue and the virus's nucleic proteins are no match for the sophistication of the human immune system including HIV. (For more information on this, I will refer you to two other books. They are *Deadly Deception*, by Dr. Robert Willner, and *Inventing the AIDS Virus*, by Peter Duesberg.)

The germs themselves are not to be feared. It is the environment that these germs grow in that allows them the strength to proliferate. "Bad germs" cannot get the upper hand on "good germs" if the tissues in which they grow are healthy and vital. It would be more constructive to think of disease and health as something that grows from within rather than something that attacks from without. This new thinking promotes building a foundation of inner support rather than attacking an outside enemy. Within the medical tenets, we should add supporting elements into dysfunctional systems to correct imbalances, deficiencies, or disharmony instead of attacking and rooting out the troubled spots.

While the four tenets of the germ theory stand as pillars in the eyes of medicine, it does not take much effort to expose the germ theory as an outdated model. If the causative germ must be present in every case of its delegated disease, how do we explain AIDS Related Complex (ARC)? After the declaration that HIV causes AIDS, medicine was confronted with people who demonstrated AIDS-like symptoms but did not have the HIV. If HIV causes AIDS, how can one exhibit the same symptoms as AIDS without the infectious virus? Either this is a brand new syndrome or AIDS does not come from HIV. Which will it be, gentlemen? You can't have it both ways. To save face and keep perpetuating the germ theory, medicine indeed created a new syndrome. AIDS Related Complex became the savior that bound this quandary to the germ theory. Though ARC resembles AIDS, it can't be AIDS because it doesn't have HIV associated with it. ARC became its own entity, though still mysteriously related to its cousin.

The second tenet of the germ theory can also be rendered false by examining something as standard as the strep throat infection. While the first tenet of the germ theory claims that germ "A" causes disease "A" every time, the second tenet of the germ theory states, therefore, that the causative germ cannot be just "hanging around doing nothing" without causing its own disease. The streptococcus bacterium is found routinely in our healthy throats. Why is it then that we are all not walking around with active, infectious strep throat? It is because Streptococcus is part of our normal cellular makeup. Cells degenerate and regenerate constantly. The streptococcus form of bacteria is part of the degenerating process of the cells. Strep throat and the abundance of streptococcus bacteria are manifested when there are more dying cells than there are regenerating cells. In other words, there is more unhealthy tissue present than there is healthy tissue. The microscopic biology has lost its homeostatic balance. You can attack the streptococcus bacteria with penicillin all you want but until the health of the throat is restored to its proper condition, "bad germs" will outnumber the "good germs." This is why our children are confronted with recurring infections. Penicillin may very well kill bacteria but is does nothing to restore the tissues of the throat (or the ear for that matter) back to a healthy state. To truly cure strep throat, the throat must revitalize to its original state of health thus keeping in balance the normal cycle of regenerating and degenerating cells.

Tenet number four of the germ theory states that the germ can be replicated and can reproduce the disease. Therefore, we are told that HIV causes AIDS and can be, as tenet number four states, transmitted through unprotected sex. Seems to fit the tenets so far. But let's reexamine tenet number one. If this was true then Magic Johnson, as well as others infected with HIV, must have signs and symptoms of AIDS. He does not.

He is very healthy. Magic Johnson does not have AIDS if he does not exhibit the signs and symptoms as defined by the condition. Herein lies an interesting snippet in the annuls of medicine. When someone defies the tenets that comprise the anointed germ theory, medicine will manipulate the definition as to perpetually promote its ideas. Tenet number four says that the germ must be able to reproduce its associated disease. HIV has not reproduced AIDS in Magic Johnson. Therefore, tenet number four does not stand the test of examination. However, to cover their tracts, medicine has delegated HIV to have stages. In magic Johnson's case The HIV simply hasn't advanced into AIDS yet. This way HIV still causes AIDS even if you do not have AIDS. But that statement now violates tenet number two which says the causative agent cannot be just "hanging around" as a germ not responsible for that disease. Can you follow that bouncing ball? Is it time now to reexamine our paradigm of health and disease or do we want to finish this book first?

Let's use some other examples. A cold sore on our upper lip caused by a virus does not spread to the lower lip but invariably the two lips touch together. Our bare feet touch together under the sheets of our bed so why doesn't our condition of athlete's foot spread from one to the other? If some people escape the dictates of the germ theory, why doesn't science focus on those individuals and examine why? Instead, they ignore these incidences pretending that these people are somehow exempt to the laws of medical science. Or better, yet, maybe people are so inclined to blind faith that they will never question the powers that be. I suppose the germ theory of disease works for everyone...except Magic Johnson...and the rest of us who do not buy into it. Any way you slice it the Germ Theory of Disease has holes in it.

We are told that mouthwash can kill the germs that cause gingivitis. The problem with this advice is that these germs are not the *cause* of gingivitis. They are the *result* of gingivitis. They are a symptom of an existing condition of decay. The condition of gingivitis creates the bacteria not the other way around. These germs are a byproduct of an unhealthy mouth. Bacteria are symbiotic scavengers. They help with the cleaning up process. They reduce dead tissue into its smallest elements. The unhealthy mouth and gums produce more decaying and dying cells than regenerating, new ones. This unhealthy condition promotes a rotten compost pile of decaying cells in your mouth. The bad germs are a product of the decaying cells. When you address the reason why the tissues that form your gums are decaying at an abnormal rate, you will stop the overload of "bad" germs. Mouthwash all you want to kill the germs that supposedly cause gingivitis but until you address the health status of the tissues in your mouth, you will constantly be rewarded with lots of "bad" germs and bad breath.

The germs and bad breath are mere byproducts of and not the cause of true gingivitis. Blaming germs for disease is akin to blaming rats and maggots for the piles of garbage in the alleyway. The garbage attracts the flies and rats in the same manner that dead tissue produces bacteria. Instead of killing the rats and flies we must remove the garbage. Instead of killing germs, we need to promote healthy tissue. We do not catch disease, we build it. Mosquitoes do not create stagnant water. They are attracted to the conditions which support their life.

Here in lies the great debate: Is it the seed or the soil? Should we focus on the germs or the tissues they grow in? Medicine wants us to focus on the seed, the germ itself, as the cause of infectious disease. They state that Streptococcus causes strep throat and germs cause gingivitis. Those schooled in Natural Law understand that our standard of health resides in the condition of the soil, your internal tissues. Nothing grows unless you feed it. That includes flowers, humans, whales, house flies, fungus, viruses, and other germs. Two corn seeds identical in every way are planted. One is planted in the rich soil of Iowa. The other is planted in the beach sand of sunny Florida. The seed planted in Iowa grows up full and strong and produces several ears of corn. The seed planted in the beach sand never cracks the earth. Why? The importance of the "seed" is minimal at best when compared to the importance of the "soil" in which it grows. This is true for germs as well as corn. It is time we put to rest the idea that germs jump on people and infect them. The only infection we are suffering from is the one in which our minds have been infected with this fallacy of germs causing disease.

A germ, isolated in a laboratory, will not grow unless you surround it with the correct media, the correct food. Stem cell research proves this very fact. Stem cells are still undifferentiated. A stem cell has not yet specialized or taken on any unique characteristics of a blood cell, bone cell, muscle cell, or whatever. When these stem cells are isolated and put into a media that stimulates bone growth they will change into osteoblasts, the precursors to mature bone. When stem cells are placed into media that stimulates red blood cells they will change into erythroblasts. The terrain stimulates the function of the cell. The vitality of the media, your tissue, will dictate whether or not germs can proliferate.

"If I could live my life over again, I would devote it to proving that germs seek their natural habitat, diseased tissue, rather than being the cause of disease."
Rudolf Virchow, father of the germ theory.

Louis Pasteur echoed similar words on his death bed. Two of the biggest names in germ hunting have recanted their own research yet medicine still marches on to the music of yesteryear.

Here is yet another conflicting point of debate. Science has tried to convince us that our genes are at fault for many of our diseases. Everything from obesity to diabetes to fibromyalgia to cancer has been implicated as being derived from a genetic defect. Even behavior is being implicated as a genetic quality. This is a scary proposition because now your neighbor is no longer responsible for molesting your child. We can blame the genes. A gambling problem is not our fault. It's our genetic makeup. We cannot control it. We have genetic tendencies to violence so we have to beat our wife. Don't believe it.

My first question is if we were not born with these conditions how do our genes just all of a sudden become defective? Are we to believe that we are having a normal life when, out of the blue, our once perfect genetic code decides to make bad muscle fibers, or a tumor, or make us act a certain way? Genes do not just decide to go bad. Once w are born with all our perfect parts in all their right places, our blueprints to all these parts, our genes, do not get erased and drawn over. They are our genes for life. We do not get one set of genes to create healthy muscle fibers and another set of genes to give us fibromyalgia later in life. We do not have one gene that creates healthy lung tissue and another one that creates emphysema. Lung tissue is lung tissue and is created from the same genetic code from conception to death.

The nucleus of the cell has long been thought of as the brain of the cell for it is here were the DNA is found. And we have been taught that it is the DNA that tells the cell how to act. I believe differently. There is another camp of thinkers and researchers that believe our genes only give us the raw materials from which to build all our parts. DNA is a warehouse of spare parts in the form of amino acids and not a brain that controls the function of the cell. The DNA does not tell the parts how to work. Nor do genes tell our parts to be dysfunctional.

Those of us who choose to look outside the dogma of the traditional establishment have found the entrenched dogma of the DNA to be misleading and outdated. Our beliefs and research, however, is silenced by the authorities in charge so you may not be aware of our contrary findings and opinions. The function of the cells, just like the germs mentioned earlier, comes from stimulus from the environment. Do you see the pattern developing here?

A cell in our body has all the functional systems that our body as a whole does. The cell has a respiratory system, a musculoskeletal system, an excretory system, a digestive system and so on. The brain of the cell is said to be located in the cell's nucleus; the DNA. Medical science tells us that the DNA gives us our spare parts in the form of amino acid building proteins. Then the DNA tells the spare parts how to act. Will it be a good gene or a defective gene? People who understand basic cellular physiology know that this is erroneous information. The DNA does not tell parts how to act like a brain directs physiology. The DNA is not the cell's brain but rather the cell's reproductive system. The DNA within the nucleus gives the cell new parts in the form of protein strands with which to build. It does not tell the parts how to function. Telling a cell how to function is the specialized role delegated to the cell membrane. The cell wall is the brain not the nucleus. This fundamental cellular physiology is taught in high school text books. However, as basic as this information is, the belief that DNA and genes dictate function is nonetheless pounded into our inquisitive minds until it becomes rote. The cellular wall has receptors which extend through it. These receptors act like antennae. The receptors perceive electromagnetic vibrational information from the environment and translate that information into the cell. It is this information that instructs the cell to change shape, move, open or close other parts of the cell's membrane, embrace the stimulus, reject the stimulus, or any number of cellular functions. For more information on this phenomenon, I would refer you to work done by Bruce Lipton.

As a carrot makes its way through the digestive process, its molecular makeup is passed into the blood for circulation. These molecules of nutrition radiate their characteristic atomic vibrational frequency. This frequency is what stimulates the cell's receptors and it is this vibrational frequency that is transmitted into the cell to create action. Cells respond to their environment. They do not dictate the environment. By applying nutrition, water, oxygen, and proper nervous stimulation (or any other form of love) to a cell membrane, we will be stimulating the cell to function in a manner in which it was designed. When the receptors detect frequencies created by physical, chemical, or emotional toxins the cell will pull away and shut down; the exact opposite of life.

A polar bear has evolved to survive in the coldness of the arctic because the environment has stimulated its genetic code to produce heavy fur and layers of fat. The polar bears eyes have specialized to adapt to the external, blinding whiteness of the snow. The external environment (macrocosm) created these changes in the bear (microcosm). In contrast, if you move the polar bear to Florida, Florida does not become cold. The bear (microcosm) does not create the environment (macrocosm). This interplay at the polar bear/external environment level is the same interaction at the DNA/cellular level. Outside, external stimulus surrounding the cell (macrocosm) will create changes within the cellular (microcosm) expression. DNA strands unwind and mold to different protein forms as this outside stimulus dictates. It is the macrocosmic external stimulus that dictates the microcosmic internal structure not the other way around.

So then, the key to avoiding harmful bacteria and

viruses does not lie in hunting them down and killing them. Nor does escaping infection rely on artificially created immunity through vaccines. Bacteria, fungus, mold, viruses, or any other form of life can only live if they find an environment that supports their existence. It makes sense then to keep our body, our soil, optimally healthy thereby prohibiting the germs, or the seeds, to grow. Creating and maintaining a healthy existence can be simplified then into the answer to this question: What elements are absolutely essential to life and consequently promote a healthy environment for our cells?

Do not be intimidated by the nature of the question. You do not need a doctoral degree to respond. In fact, that is exactly the point of this book.

You will not need to submerge yourself in a quagmire of textbooks and internet surfing. The answer is not complicated at all. Our cells, whether they are part of our brain, eyelashes, pancreas, bone marrow, colon, or any other part of us need only four forms of stimulus to exist in a healthy state. They need proper nutrition, water, oxygen, and an animating energy source.

Chiropractors call this animating energy innate intelligence and it flows through the nervous system. Acupuncturists call this energy chi and it flows through pathways called meridians. God calls this energy love and it flows through nature. Call it what you will but that's it! Food, water, oxygen, and an energizing impetus to control and regulate the cell's functions are the only stimulus needed to maintain health. Whether we are concerned with one cell or you as an entire human being, these are the elements essential to life. No more can you stop the rain from falling, stop the birds from migrating, or stop the earth from quaking than you can stop these four essentials from stimulating health.

Every human also needs sunshine and rest but these two elements are more passive. The sun always shines and all we need to do is go outside and enjoy its health benefits. And the body will not let us stay awake forever. It will eventually make us sleep. It is here, in deep sleep that our body will repair, regenerate, and heal. Sleeping disorders can be helped by addressing the first four essentials listed prior.

Every cell in our body and every body on this planet require proper nutrition, water, oxygen, and a self-regulating energy source/nervous system to exist. Life does not depend on processed sugar, hydrogenated fats, $3,000.00 designer purses, cigarettes, cell phones, allergy medicine, a gas guzzling SUV, or Ibuprophen to survive. Life does not require hormone replacement therapy, the Super Bowl, nasal decongestants, inhalers, or music television to exist. If it did, we would all be required to receive these additives to our daily regimen. But we don't. The only elements absolutely 100% needed for survival, I will reiterate, are nutrition, water, oxygen, and an animating energy source/ your nervous system.

Try and go without food, water, air, or your nervous system and see what happens. Stop breathing right now. How long can we go without air? The average person will have three to five minutes. How long can we go without food? If we did not put another bite of food in our mouth we could watch our body wither away and eventually die within 30 to 45 days. Every piece of our cells, every hormone in our body, every chemical in our brain, every neurotransmitter, every blood vessel, muscle fiber, every digestive enzyme, every piece of bone, every last inch of our packaging is built directly from the nutrition that we feed our self. Where else would these parts come from? They do not just magically appear out of thin air. If we insist on eating junk food and processed, refined, instant, prepackaged foods, our body will give it all back to us in the same form of useless, ineffective body parts. How long can we go without water? The statistics say seven to ten days. The fact that these elements are essential to supporting life means something. Ignore them and we will feel the results in the form of some illness, disease, or premature degeneration.

Last but certainly not least, when we cross our leg over our other knee while sitting, what happens to the sensation in our leg? Our fibula bone, the thin bone running along the outside of our lower leg, compresses the peroneal nerve causing our leg to fall asleep. Our leg is being deprived of its energy source via the nervous system. What if we go beyond compression and cut the nerve off completely? Only one thing can happen and that is paralysis. Without a nerve supply there is no human life. With reduced nerve supply there is reduced human life.

When it comes to life, health, and our very existence, these are the only four tangible items that we need. Cut them out of our life completely and we will die. Limit their potential to support us properly and we will not face imminent death but we will suffer premature degeneration and become more susceptible to illness and disease. That's it. That's the answer to health care. It is that simple.

Within the new world view of quantum physics, one could argue that we humans need a positive, nurturing sense of belonging. We all need the energy of love. Love is the energetic glue that holds all the life sustaining, electromagnetic, vibrational frequencies together. For those of us who need to focus on the tangible elements of nutrition, water, oxygen and a nervous system, we can just as easily remain grounded without the complexities of existentialism. Remember that Einstein proved that matter is energy and energy is matter, so by making changes at the physical level we can create changes within the energetic, spiritual level without the awkward feeling that this "new age" talk of energy may conjure up. Feeding our body its required physical needs is, by virtue of quantum physics, feeding our body the same energy of love. The spirit of medicine needs a revival and we can start by relearning how to love our self by respecting and feeding our body what it needs.

There is no magic bullet and no fountain of youth. I realize that can be a hard pill for many people to swallow but like most Americans, we have swallowed tons of pills prior to reading this book so one more won't hurt. We are constantly reminded that we cannot survive without prescription drugs. We are bombarded with ads every day on the television, radio, and in the newspapers and magazines that remind us that we cannot achieve an erection, breath the springtime air, eat certain foods, concentrate, have a regular menstrual cycle, or even sleep properly without being medicated. We will all die from skin cancer if we do not use sun screen. Having a common emotion like sadness may be a sign of depression and that needs medical attention. We are reminded of the epidemics that will spread if we do not keep to our vaccination schedules. These kinds of fear based statements are designed to promote dependency on medication. We are incessantly being made aware of our imperfect bodies that cannot cope with life's natural processes and invariably will need copious amounts of intervention. This indoctrination, brainwashing in a sense, is just that. It is one way of thinking and only one way of thinking. We have the choice right now to change our way of thinking and change our life.

In the following chapters, I will discuss nutrition, water, oxygen, and animating energy as they relate to chiropractic, acupuncture, whole food supplements, exercise, and better lifestyle choices. I will show you how they fit into the quantum physics model of holism as they all provide nourishment to the entire body, mind, and spirit. By implementing these simple recommendations, we can become healthier, attain a higher quality of life, decrease dependency on drugs, and increase awareness of our own perfection.

"Live each season as it passes, breathe the air, drink the drink, taste the fruit, and resign yourself to the influences of each."
Henry David Thoreau

CHAPTER EIGHT

YOU ARE WHAT YOU EAT

"Let your food be your medicine and your medicine be your food."
    Hippocrates

There is only one reason why we need to eat. There are many reasons why we do eat: to satisfy a craving, to bury an emotional uprising, to be social, or even just because we are bored, but there is only one reason why we *need* to eat. That is so the food can be broken down and digested to provide nutrition to our cells. Period. That is it. Everything else is just filler. Everything we do from selecting which foods to eat, to choosing the method of preparation, to chewing, and ultimately to swallowing, are all geared toward only one end result. As we feed ourselves, we feed our cells. The food we take in is ultimately converted into energy, building materials, and nutrition for our cells so they can do their job as efficiently as possible. Though our eyes and taste buds may most assuredly be deceiving us, when our stomach rumbles it is not asking for a fast food burrito whose meat filling is comprised mostly of lard. It is asking for fats, proteins, carbohydrates, vitamins, minerals and enzymes from live food to convert into real living breathing tissue.

The communication systems of our bodies are requesting real food in the form of oranges, kidney beans, and cucumbers. Our body knows no other language. It was encoded at birth with all the necessary equipment to make its way through this world. We were given eyes to see, lungs to breathe, and legs to walk.

Each specific part joins together to make us a whole person. This teamwork is nothing short of miraculous. This biological wonder knows instinctively how to take care of itself. Nobody had to show our circulatory system how to form a clot when we are cut. It already knew how to carry the protein thromboplastin through four stages of reactions involving some 13 different factors and eventually creating a final mesh like protein called fibrin. Our liver did not need to go to college to learn the puzzling diagram outlining the Kreb's cycle and the electron transport chain. It had been converting glucose into energy long before man even had a written language. When it comes to nutritional needs, our body does not lose its sense of intrinsic know how. The same wisdom it uses to continuously blink your eyes to keep them moist calls for life supporting vitamins, minerals and enzymes found only in live, real food.

If we were to build a house and we opted to use termite infested wood, bent nails, frayed wiring, rusted piping, and broken window panes, how long would that house last? Would it keep us safe and warm? If the framework of this house came under any kind of stress, like a pounding thunder storm, would it be able to stand up to the added pressure? Our body responds in the same manner. If we feed it with second rate nutrition, if we supply it with substandard parts from which to build the housing of our body, we will suffer the same consequences. We will be weak and unable to stand up to the rigors of daily living. We will be much more susceptible to breaking down. We will wear out prematurely. The medical community is the only successful business that does not understand the value of using quality raw materials to build quality structure. Have they ever promoted the use of organic whole foods as a preventative to disease? What separates a BMW from a Yugo? Quality. What's the difference between a five star restaurant and the fast food restaurant chain found on every corner? Quality. One of the factors in the difference between health and disease, life and death, is the quality of the food we consume.

This violation of feeding is not unique to the human form. Mad cow disease has evolved from a practice of feeding the herds in a manner contrary to nature's design. Science deemed it a safe practice to turn the world's herbivorous cows into carnivorous meat eaters. Cows are designed to graze on grasses yet the agriculture authorities allow farmers to feed their cows slaughterhouse waste. This direct violation of Natural Law and its food chain has its consequences. Mad cow disease is not some mysterious virus from the tropical rain forest or an alien bacterium from Mars attacking these poor innocent cows. It is a prion, an infectious protein that is responsible for the mayhem. We have turned our cows into cannibals. Cows are not carnivores. Never have been and never will be. The cow's digestive system is not programmed to handle animal protein. When it is faced with this task, the system is sent into a state of confusion. The resulting attempt to process this foreign matter is a build-up of toxic metabolites that scramble the cow's brain. What could we possible expect when we completely ignore nature's rules and feed grass grazing creatures anything other than what grows in the pasture? What can we expect from humans when we are filled with bleached foods, preservatives, hydrogenated fats, artificial colors, and processed sugars? The answer...a less than perfect, mutated life form just like our mad cows.

  Our cells can only perform to the level of nutrition they receive. If we are stuffed with greasy fast food, sugar laden soda, artificially flavored and colored potato chips, hydrogenated oils, preservatives, pesticides, and processed, bleached flour, how on earth can we expect our cells to give us back anything but that in return? Our body has no choice but to try its best and manifest health through a fog of nutritional insufficiency and deficiency. We will become, in time, a walking, talking, breathing donut stuffed-french fried-chocolate covered-ice cream filled-cola soaked bag of carbon molecules. This is basic human digestive physiology. Garbage in, garbage out. If we consume bad fats, our body will make unhealthy brain tissue which will lead to poor memory, ADD, sluggish thinking, depression, and a foggy sense of being. We would never exchange high octane premium gasoline for leaded gasoline when it comes to fueling a Porsche. Our body is no different. Would we expect our body's engine to respond better to a broccoli salad or to the high fructose corn syrup found in soda, bottled iced teas, and other assorted fruit drinks? We are, after all, exactly what we eat.

If our cells are not fed properly they will pull calcium and other minerals from our bones. Our muscle tissue will be broken down for protein. Other organs will be called upon to reinforce or substitute for another ailing organ or system. In time this neglect will catch up with us. Mark my words. Heart disease, high cholesterol, osteoporosis, type II diabetes, high blood pressure, obesity, arteriosclerosis, and allergies all have a direct link to chronically poor food choices. It is these diseases that are currently some of the biggest challenges to the medical community. Let us add to that list fibromyalgia, psoriasis, irritable bowel, sinusitis, chronic fatigue, and ADD. Each of these conditions can be greatly improved upon with better decision making concerning our selections of food. In fact, any and every condition can only improve when better food choices are selected. That is Universal Law dictated from a divine order.

The bittersweet tale to our nightmarish food choices is that after all the junk we stuff into ourselves, our brilliant anatomy and physiology manage somehow to wake us up in the morning and get us on our feet. Our body finds a way to pull out whatever minuscule semblance of nutrition we give it and keeps us alive. Our body compensates. If we do not provide the needed nutrition, our body will pull what it needs from your tissues and organs. If we do not supply ourselves with enough zinc, our body will draw from the cellular storage in the prostate. Over a period of time this will weaken the prostate and leave it susceptible to disease.

Have you ever questioned why the flu season attacks the population in the winter time? Why isn't the government sending the flu-mobile to your neighborhood in the summer time? The virility of the flu bug has nothing to do with the temperature fluctuations of the seasons. We do not succumb to the flu because we did not wear a hat in the cold air. We cannot blame our coworkers for giving us the bug. One only needs to examine the fall and winter holidays to quickly determine the grounds by which the flu relegates itself to the cold weather. We start off the season in October with Halloween in which we stuff our children and ourselves full of processed sugar in the form of trick or treat candy. No sooner has their immune system been assaulted with an overload of sugar when we are confronted with Thanksgiving. Sweet potatoes baked in brown sugar, cranberry sauce, wine, followed up with cookies and pies will add to the already sugar burdened immune system. But do not worry. Just around the corner are Christmas, Hanukkah and New Years. More celebration, more parties, more sugar laden foods. Have we had enough? Wait. February is fast approaching and that means Valentines Day with more chocolate candy. *Processed sugar is not food!* It is a foreign substance and the body will mount an immune attack to fight it off. Not only is the immune system over burdened through this season of sugar overload but the sugar will effectively strip our bodies of the already depleted minerals stores needed to protect us from infection. On top of that we can add a flu shot but the flu shot only adds more toxins to our struggling body. (More about vaccines later.) Our best bet in avoiding the wintertime flu is to vastly decrease the sugar intake and conversely increase our intake of foods rich in vitamin A, C, and E. Does that seem too simple to believe?

The degree to which our health improves will

depend on many other variables. One such variable is the intensity by which we attend to our dietary insufficiencies. If we only add one banana at breakfast to our daily routine and we continue to consume large amounts of refined white flour products, chances are we may not see or feel any appreciable difference in our health. We will improve our health only to the magnitude in which we change all bad habits. When we decide to add flaxseed oil to our regimen to help with the stiffness associated with arthritis but we do not discontinue drinking dark colas (the overload of phosphoric acid from the colas will leach the calcium from your bones) we will be defeating the whole purpose of adding flaxseed. We cannot be half hearted about our nutritional decisions and expect whole hearted results. If we do what we did, we get what we got. Nothing will change until we make the changes. The decision to be sick or healthy is one only we can make.

We all know that from the day we are born there will come a day when we take our last breath. The time we spend in between those two events does not have to be filled with degenerative, chronic suffering. We can age gracefully and with some dignity. We can look forward to our senior years with a sense of excitement and not frustration. Eating the proper foods now is a retirement program for our future. We initially do not see the labors of our investment but as we come closer to cashing in this nutritional IRA, we will be quite surprised as to the benefits we will reap.

For example, let us look briefly at heart disease, clogged arteries, and arteriosclerosis. Co-Q10 increases oxygenation of the heart tissue. Vitamin E improves circulation, promotes normal blood clotting, reduces blood pressure, strengthens the capillaries, prevents cell damage, and reduces scarring. Garlic is one of the most valuable foods on the planet. Its medicinal qualities have been recorded as far back as ancient Babylonia. Garlic can help lower blood pressure, reduces the chance of blood clots by inhibiting the platelet from sticking together, lowers cholesterol, is a natural antibiotic, and an immune stimulant. Anyone suffering from heart disease, clogged arteries, or arteriosclerosis will benefit from a diet rich in fatty fish such as salmon. Eggs, nuts and seeds, wheat germ, cold pressed extra virgin olive oil, and dark green leafy vegetables also aid in supplying nutrition for a healthy cardiovascular system. We must also avoid hydrogenated oils and discontinue consuming products containing caffeine. Instead of our doctors educating us on this aspect of heart health care, we are told that taking an aspirin a day can benefit our hearts. Will we become an aspirinaholic? It sounds like the blood thinning ability of aspirin is once again chasing those elusive symptoms. Is your blood really too thick and is in need of thinning or is your cardiovascular system clogged with indigestible, non-nutritional pieces of left over sludge?

    Dr. Dean Ornish pioneered and revolutionized cardiovascular care by proving nutrition has an undeniable cause and effect action on heart health. How many of you now are saying Dr Who? That's exactly my point. He proved that heart disseminated to the public. As long as I continue to see aspirin therapy promoted on television for cardiovascular health instead of Dr. Dean Ornish's recommendations and Mother Nature's healing foods I must stand on the mountain top and scream, "Stop the madness!" disease could be reversed not with the use of drugs but with proper food choices and lifestyle changes. This kind of information should be embraced by the medical community and immediately

    High cholesterol can be addressed with the addition of red yeast rice to the diet which is a fermentation byproduct of cooked non-glutinous rice. Though red yeast rice is a common food source in China, it is most often found here in supplement form. (Since I began writing this book, the FDA has found it necessary to stop the sale of red yeast rice on some trumped up political charge. The truth of the matter is that too many people were benefiting from it and prescriptions for cholesterol medications were declining). Oat bran, flaxseed, garlic, wheat germ, and black currant seed also play a role in a healthy cholesterol balance. Calcium in the form of green vegetables such as broccoli and Brussels sprouts is another good preventative therapy for elevated cholesterol levels. But again, we must stop the poor decision making that got us where we are in the first place. I can live without Lipitor. It is not essential to life. I cannot live without proper nutrition that supports the appropriate functioning of my cells.

Here is another example. Diabetics will benefit from adding brewer's yeast, brown rice, whole grains, and blackstrap molasses to their diet as those foods can supply important chromium and other trace minerals needed in the producing of insulin. Keep in mind that a diabetic does not just have a sick pancreas and poor insulin production. Every cell in their body feels the effects of these nutritional deficiencies. The entire digestive system, and ultimately the entire body, is suffering. The pancreas works in concert with the gall bladder, liver, stomach and other digestive organs. When one member of the team does not fulfill its obligations, the others must find some way to compensate for the lack of cooperation. Every one of the organs suffer. This is true for any illness, syndrome, or disease. Supporting the liver with Spanish black radish and betaine from beets is important as well as adding inositol from brewer's yeast. Enzymes from avocados, papayas, pineapples, mangos, and sprouts are powerful adjuncts to any digestive disorder. This is not a cure all diet for diabetes. It is a recommendation to reevaluate the level of one's health and its relationship to better food choices.

While agencies have instituted RDA's for vitamins, fiber, amino acids, calcium, magnesium and other minerals, you will never find an RDA for Prevacid or any other drug. RDA stands for recommended dietary allowance. Science has created a guideline for establishing the minimal quantities of certain elements needed in our diet each day. We absolutely need to take in vitamins A, B, C, D, E and K, and the minerals calcium, zinc, potassium, sodium, and selenium as well as other nutrients. If we neglect these nutritives, deficiencies will manifest and pathologies will arise. We can surf the internet for eons of time, we can scour the shelves of the biggest libraries, but we will never find an RDA for Celebrex, Tagamet, Coumadin, or Flexeril. When did Naprosyn, Claritin, Zoloft, and Ritalin become part of our everyday diets? Have you ever seen their pictures in the food pyramid? Of course not. That is because they are not essential to life. They are not needed to supply our bodies with required vitamins and minerals.

"When I tell the truth, it is not for the sake of convincing those who do not know it, but for the sake of defending those that do."
William Blake

It is easy to make fun of folk medicine. We can conger up images of witches gathered around a cauldron while they mix up a potion. We can laugh at the Amish family that eats raw onion and garlic to cure a cold. Instead of assuming that folk medicine is archaic and those who practice it are just plain weird, we might wonder whether there is some justification in their actions. The origin of pharmaceuticals has its roots lodged in folk remedies and natural sources. Pharmaceutical companies cannot patent, and therefore make profits on, natural phenomena so they have to synthesize nature's perfection and mass produce a chemical wannabe version of it.

Valium is a synthetic derivative of the root of the

valerian plant. Valerian root has been used for eons of time to reduce stress, anxiety, and insomnia. It is a natural sedative. Valium became the man made version, the artificial form, of valerian root. Only in this form can it be patented, mass produced, and promoted as just what the doctor ordered. Aspirin was created by the pharmaceutical companies to mass produce a synthetic form of salicylic acid. Willow bark, which contains natural salicylic acid, had been used by aboriginal people to ease the pain associated with body aches for centuries. The latest generation of anti- inflammatory drugs is COX-2 inhibitors in the form of Celebrex and Vioxx. Bromelain from pineapple, quercetin from eucalyptus, curcumin from turmeric, and boswellia have been doing the same thing ever since God put them on our earth. Synthetic Digitalis, a medicine for heart failure, originated from foxglove. The poppy flower gave us morphine. Not only can foods, herbs, and plants be used medicinally, they have none of the dangerous side effects of synthetic supplements or pharmaceuticals. They work *with* the body to build life not *against* the body to artificially control function.

    Ironically, medical doctors will offer us their own version of the witch's brew. Drug companies disguise it as science and sell it in the form of pharmaceuticals. For example, Premarin is a form of estrogen therapy for post menopausal women. Its name is derived from combining the three words from which are the source of the drug; pregnant mare's urine. How exactly is that supposed to nourish the body's cells? Premarin has been reported to increase the risk of endometrial cancer. Synthetic estrogen replacement therapy has been implicated in an increased risk of breast cancer. Is ridding hot flashes with pregnant mare's urine worth the risk of endometrial or breast cancer? I guarantee that none of us have a deficiency of pregnant mare's urine. However, complimenting the diet with wheat germ oil, wild yam, ginseng, cod liver oil, or the herbs black cohosh and tribulus will make the transition from motherhood to a keeper of wisdom much more tolerable and graceful. Doesn't that sound more inviting and nurturing than a mouthful of pregnant mare's urine and high risk cancer groups?

Our body's immune system has the ability to distinguish between helpful bacteria and harmful ones. It can detect an invading virus or foreign body and mount an impressive immune response to create antibodies. That same inborn intelligence exists in every system and every cell of our body. This includes the digestive system which knows the difference between real butter and plastic margarine. It will accept, without hesitation, the nutrition pulled from a grape, a salmon fillet, and kale. It knows just exactly how to change a tomato and a pinto bean into flesh and blood without the approval of the FDA. Our body's wisdom can appreciate the life giving qualities of parsley and cashews and convert them into its own expression of life even if the AMA does not value them. The divine know how of our anatomy will recognize MSG, sodium nitrate, and bleached flour as non-foods and attack them the same way it does any other foreign invader despite the food processing companies' propaganda. They are not food. They are foreign invaders and do not possess any sustainable qualities.

We have devitalized our food sources to such a point that we now have health food marketed as a specialty. How preposterous! All real food in its natural whole state is healthy. Why does real food need that label?

The very name "health food" infers that other supermarket food items are not healthy. We should drop the stigma "health food", as by its own inherent nature food is healthy, and then label processed items as "junk food." The grocery stores have entire aisles reserved for soda, cookies, and chips. In contrast, there may be a few shelves or an end cap of granola bars and organic products. So-called health food is just real food and real food feeds and nourishes our cells. Cells that are nourished in the manner consistent with the Big Picture will function properly and remain in a state of health. It is that simple.

Our body is waiting to be filled with fresh water, bananas, apples, green peas, and sweet potatoes. No matter what brainwashing we receive from the media, the plain simple fact is that our body requires real, unadulterated food in its natural state to maintain itself in a position of optimal health. From this, it can assimilate the proper nutrition for biological function. Our body does so without the knowledge of text books or guidance from a dietician. Anything less and we have bought ourselves a one way ticket to the doctor's office. We can feed our body pears, squash, eggplant, and zucchini or we can poison it with over processed, man-made food like high fructose corn syrup, aspartame, hydrogenated oils, and toxic medicinals. We are solely responsible for the decisions we make concerning food choices. Do we opt for longevity, clarity of mind, grace and dignity with aging, wisdom, and a sense of spiritual connectedness or do we choose to live out our final decades riddled with arthritis, diabetes, heart disease, cancer, or some other debilitating illness?

"If it grows, eat it. If it doesn't grow, don't eat it."
Louise Hay

CHAPTER NINE

MILK, CALCIUM, OSTEOPOROSIS, AND ALLERGIES

"If the Lord delight in us, then he will bring us into this land, and give it us; a land which floweth with milk and honey."
Numbers 14:8

We cannot go a day without being confronted with some advertisement concerning calcium and strong bones. We are continually reminded that "milk does a body good" and "TUMS is fortified with calcium." We have seen the celebrities sporting milk mustaches in our favorite magazines. Many of our foods now come fortified with calcium and they are proud to brag about it on the packaging: orange juice, crackers, pancake mix, and breakfast cereals to name a few. By looking at the shelf of vitamins in our local supermarket or drug store, we will see a wide variety of calcium supplementation available to us. There is calcium citrate, lactate, carbonate, coral calcium, gluconate, calcium chloride, as well as oyster shell and bone meal. We oblige these pleas for calcium intake by consuming dairy products; cheese, ice cream, and milk at the rate of nearly 600 pounds per person each year.[5]

With all this availability and consumption of calcium, why does osteoporosis affect 28 million Americans?[6] Well, let's start by blaming soda for all this osteoporosis. We have to blame someone, right? The research says today's children are drinking more soda (and conversely less milk) which puts them at a greater

---

[5] Morrison, E.M. "Dairy's New Design." April-June 2005. Agricultural Utilization Research Institute.
<http://www.auri.org/news/aniapr05/mncommoditiesdairy.htm>
[6] American Academy of Orthopaedic Surgeons.
http://orthoinfo:aaos.org

risk for developing osteoporosis. The phosphoric acid in soda leeches calcium from our bones. The amount of sugar that is put into a can of soda is grossly negligent and can interfere with the hormones that regulate calcium in the body. (Sugar substitutes have their own set of health warnings and issues.) And, because refined sugar is void of nutrients/minerals, it actually pulls minerals from the tissues as it passes through the body. (Remember physics taught us that nature hates a vacuum/void.) Though these facts hold merit for today's generation, they do not take into account my parent's and grandparent's generation of bone thinning conditions before soda was consumed on such a massive scale.

Maybe we can blame Dr. Spock, the world's pre-eminent and most trusted pediatrician as he has influenced generations of mothers with his book, *Baby and Child Care.* Selling more than 50 million copies, its popularity has become ubiquitous. He recommended that no one drink cow's milk at any age. Dr. Spock associated milk drinking with heart disease, cancer, obesity, asthma, and ear infections. Cow's milk is one of the biggest contributors to childhood allergies. Milk is also a predominant factor in chronic ear infections. Stop consuming dairy products and these health issues, if not completely resolved, will be greatly improved.

Regardless of Dr. Spock's advice, Milk consumption is at an all time high. Didn't we all grow up drinking three glasses of milk every day? I know my contemporaries were practically force fed milk by school programs and mothers who only wanted to do what they thought was best for their children. So why all the osteoporosis?

Science loves to do research to prove its point of view but when the research falls short of that goal it will become buried in a pile of bureaucracy. Have you ever heard of the 12 year study at Harvard concerning osteoporosis which involved nearly 78,000 women? This is a prestigious university and an enormous control group that required earth to complete twelve trips around the sun. The result? Come on, you've heard the conclusion haven't you? No? It wasn't on the front page of your daily newspaper? It wasn't headlining the nightly news? It was published in the *American Journal of Public Health* in 1997 but who reads that? The conclusion was that women who got the most dairy calcium actually suffered more fractures than women who got little or none. The National Institute of Health published similar findings in *The American Journal of Clinical Nutrition* (2001) as did the University of Sydney and Westmead Hospital in their publication found in *The American Journal of Epidemiology* (1994). The milk debate continues in *Pediatrics* (2003) stating, "A cautious approach demands taking milk's risks seriously and providing other beverage choices." In 2001, *The American Journal of Clinical Nutrition* asked, "Why do populations who consume low-calcium diets have fewer fractures than do those with high intakes?"

Yale University did us all a favor when they reviewed 34 published studies in 16 countries. The combined conclusion was that those countries with the highest rates of osteoporosis, including the United States, Finland, and Sweden, are those in which people consume the most dairy. The Physicians Committee for Responsible Medicine agrees and they include the likes of Dean Ornish, Andrew Weil, and John McDougall; all well known leaders in their field.

So why is there such a discrepancy? If we consume such large quantities of calcium enriched foods which should enhance our bone strength, why do we also have epidemic proportions of bone thinning disease? There are several reasons (including the overconsumption of soda mentioned above.) Here again, science's quest for minimalism has isolated one aspect of the magnificent complex we call bone. Though calcium may be the main constituent of bone and gives bone its mass, it does not give bone its strength. The bone matrix is held together by an array of trace minerals such as boron, silica, copper, phosphorous, magnesium, zinc, manganese and others. Another study published in the January 2000, *American Journal of Clinical Nutrition*, backs up my point by stating that the nutrients in fruits and vegetables (potassium, beta-carotene, vitamin C, magnesium) were associated with higher bone density. It is these trace minerals that become the glue within the calcium. They combine with the calcium in forming a strong skeletal system.

To single out calcium deficiency as the sole cause of osteoporosis is like saying Michael Jordan is the only reason the Chicago Bulls won six world championships. It is true that while they both play major roles in their respective capacities, they are not, by any means, the whole story. For each to succeed they need assistance. Calcium has the trace minerals to support its integrity and Michael Jordan had his teammates to chip in and contribute. No man is an island and no bone is just calcium. Strength and success lie in a cooperation of a synergistic resonance. Each piece of the puzzle plays a vital role in the make-up of the whole. With all this focus on calcium we have forgotten to fortify our bones with trace minerals.

Another reason for the massive discrepancy in calcium consumption and osteoporosis is that calcium, in and of itself, is not readily absorbed through the digestive process. Its bioavailability, its capability to be utilized at a cellular level, depends on help from other select nutrients. (Can you see a theme of teamwork starting?) Just supplying calcium, or any other nutrient, into our body does not equate a reaction at the cellular level and it is here were the magic happens. Unless our body properly processes the nutrition to work within the cells, it is utterly useless. The nutrition will pass through and be eliminated without being absorbed. For calcium to be properly and efficiently absorbed we need to combine it with magnesium, vitamin D, phosphorous, and essential fatty acids.

If we have come to believe that popping antacids would not only soothe our heartburn but also provide us with calcium, we have been misled. Calcium is best assimilated and absorbed when initially exposed to an acidic digestive system; That being found in the stomach. Calcium carbonate, the calcium found in antacids, is used to *decrease* stomach acid production. This is counteractive to Natural Law and to what is needed to begin the process of producing a bioavailable, ionized form of calcium that can interact at a cellular level. Our stomach needs to be acidic to break down and create a usable form of calcium and antacids will not accomplish that task.

Calcium carbonate is a hard, inorganic form of calcium that needs to transfer through nearly a dozen chemical reactions before it can be reconstructed into a usable form of calcium. This calcium, found in the earth, cannot be digested by the body. It is in an inorganic form. Humans are not designed to eat dirt. The plants have the ability to utilize this inorganic calcium and turn it into organic calcium lactate. That is the calcium we humans can digest. Plant based calcium is organic, perfectly digestible, and exactly what we are designed to eat. We are not plants and therefore cannot change inorganic calcium into organic calcium. We need broccoli, kale, okra, spinach and the like to do that for us.

What about some other form of calcium supplementation that is not in an antacid? Check the back of the bottle for the source of the calcium. Most companies use calcium carbonate due to its inexpensive availability. It is cheap to market. It does contain a higher ratio of calcium than other sources but may be the least effective. Remember, quantity does not equate quality. Calcium carbonate is chalk no matter what label is put on it. So what is your calcium supplement source? Calcium lactate is vegetable based calcium and is the kind of calcium our bodies can use.

Improperly processed bone meal and dolomite are two other poor choices when it comes to selecting your supplements. They, like oyster shell and limestone, are hard inorganic forms of calcium. The bone meal and dolomite have also been found to contain lead, mercury, and other contaminants.

A purist will argue that cow's milk was designed and perfected by nature to help baby calves grow into big cows. It has the unmitigated distinction of the perfect blend of vitamins, minerals, fats, and proteins to get that specific job done. Feline milk is engineered to turn little kittens into big cats. Elephants have their own recipe for complimenting the growth of their babies as well. There are more than 4,000 different species of milk drinking mammals and each one has its own unique needs when it comes to newborns and nursing mothers. Each species claims the exact blend of colostrum, antibodies, amino acids, lactose, fatty acids, vitamins, and minerals to create their own unique formula to rear that specific species. Mother's breast milk, regardless of the species, is the only milk source their babies will ever need. If nature designed us mammals to consume milk throughout our entire lives, we would all, horses, dogs, raccoons, humans and the like, still be latched onto dear old mom. However, you never see that amongst our animal relatives. Nature knows when enough is enough. Mammals instinctively wean their young from the breast at a certain age. It is nature's way of saying that the child has had enough breast milk and is ready to eat solid food.

Least we not forget that human mother's breast milk is sterile. By forcing industrial cow's milk into our babies we are also contaminating our children with a slew of bovine growth hormones, antibiotics, bovine vaccines, and any pesticide residue found in the cow's food. None of these are indigenous to the human diet.

Consuming indigestible forms of calcium can

lead to calcium deficiencies as the body cannot properly utilize the source. Symptoms of which include depression, hypertension, insomnia, cramping pain, nervousness, numbness in the extremities, aching joints, and heart palpitations. People who oppose nutritional supplements claim we should get all our nutrition from the foods we eat. That is absolutely correct. It is the ideal. Unfortunately, it is a rarity indeed to find a household with organic raw food bounding from the refrigerator. Organic foods can only supply needed nutrition if you eat them. It is a great way to maintain a healthy state. If one finds themselves, however, in a state of illness, therapeutic doses of certain nutritive's may be needed. To obtain a therapeutic level of calcium, or any other nutritionally based deficiency, a supplement is highly recommended. My personal choice of supplements will be discussed later in the book.

Now we may be questioning just exactly where are we supposed to get our calcium from if not from dairy products? Calcium lactate, the calcium found in green leafy vegetables such as asparagus, broccoli, cabbage, kale, kelp, dulse, mustard greens, and turnip greens is the most easily digested form of calcium. It is an organic food based source. A salad of mixed greens is a wonderful source of calcium. Other foods such as blackstrap molasses, brewer's yeast, figs, oats, and prunes offer a calcium source that can be used by the body. We can get calcium from nuts such as almonds, walnuts, hazelnuts, and sunflower seeds. Herbs that contain calcium are alfalfa, fennel seed, flaxseed, parsley, paprika, and chamomile.

Now here's the catch and this is where I stand on the great milk debate: Do we or do we not drink cow's milk? Though I do certainly agree we should all eat more vegetables, I have to consider that (and I give lots of credence to) our aboriginal ancestors. They drank milk and ate butter, yogurt, kefir, and cheese. Are hundreds of years of intuitive behavior wrong?

The difference between their dairy products and

the dairy products we consume today is pasteurization. Generations before us did not pasteurize milk. It was raw. The pasteurization process heats the milk to kill dangerous bacteria. Dangerous bacteria in milk only became a problem as we industrialized farms. Dirty crowded industrial farms have a greater potential to create sick cows that produce yucky milk filled with pus and dangerous bacteria.

In all the years of listening to my parents and grandparents retelling the stories of their youth, stories of the dairy farms and fresh milk delivery, I never once heard them say, "But you had to be so careful with raw milk. Kids were getting sick and dying. It was an epidemic." Those were the days when people took pride in producing a quality product. Farmer's names were attached to the milk. Can you imagine what would happen to the reputation of Farmer John if word got out that people were getting sick from his milk? His family would go hungry because his business would fail. Most of today's farms are corporate owned or controlled. There's no name attached to them. It's Big Agra with deep pockets. The more milk the sell, the more money they make.

"Get off your horse and drink your milk."
John Wayne

Where cows used to roam the pasture, eat lush green grass, soak in the sunshine and fresh air (health clean cows produce healthy clean milk), they are now confined to overcrowded stalls, are force fed corn as cows are natural grass eaters, and are shot up with antibiotics, steroids, and rBGH to increase milk production. Cows treated with growth hormones (rBGH) require more energy-dense food. This has usually been provided as meat and bone meal derived from rendered animals. Cows are herbivores. They are not supposed to eat other animal parts. This act of feeding has been implicated in the cause of mad cow disease. So which scenario's milk needs to be sterilized?

This heating process of pasteurization also changes the entire chemical makeup of the milk. Remember your days in chemistry class? What does heat do to the structure of molecules? When heat is added to a molecule, the binding elements of the molecule expand causing distortion, and most likely will break thus making a new arrangement of atoms.

The proteins congeal, the enzymes are burned off (we need the enzyme lactase to breakdown lactose!) and the vitamins are destroyed. Then we scoop out all the cream and add homogenization. The stuff you buy in the grocery store resembles nothing like what came out of the cow originally.

In my opinion, pasteurized milk is nothing more than poisonous sugar water. How many people do you know (maybe even yourself) who are allergic or sensitive to dairy or even lactose intolerant? How many people are now confined to drinking Lactaid, soy milk, rice milk, or almond milk because their digestive systems have rebuked pasteurized milk?

While most countries give consumers the option of drinking raw or pasteurized milk, (According to the regulations in the European Union all raw milk products are legal and considered safe for human consumption) most states in this country, unfortunately, have made it illegal to sell unpasteurized milk in grocery stores. You must find a food co-op or farm near you. www.realmilk.com can help.

A classic book in the field of health and natural medicine, *Nutrition and Physical Degeneration*, written by Weston Price, discusses the health benefits and absolute necessity of the consumption of raw milk and high vitamin butter oil by our ancestral tribes. Their use of these products was always in a pure, natural, unadulterated form.

Weston Price traveled the world in the 1940s and studied indigenous diets. He found several factors common to all tribes and clans. One of these was the consumption of raw, whole milk. The intuitive nature of man knew that raw, whole milk had healing qualities that are essential to proper growth and health.

Other than the obvious calcium and protein, raw unpasteurized milk from grass fed cows delivers iron, magnesium, phosphorus, selenium, chromium, iodine, copper, zinc, sodium, and manganese. Saturated fat and cholesterol, two very controversial (due to bad science) but extremely essential substances, are found in every cell membrane in our bodies. Raw milk supplies them to us. Lactoferrin (assists in the absorption of iron), a multitude of enzymes including lysozyme (antibiotic arsenal that can kill bad bacteria), and vitamins A and D can round out the ingredients. The nutritive content can vary of course depending on many factors.

My grandparents and parents had fresh milk and other dairy products delivered to their house every day. The difference between then and now is that our milk today is pasteurized, homogenized, skimmed, and chemically dismantled. It resembles nothing like the milk our ancestors drank. It is my opinion that dairy products from grass fed cows are not dangerous if they are served in a whole, raw, organic, natural state and consumed in moderation. There are two sides to every story including the debate on dairy foods. If you have health care concerns, pasteurized dairy products may be a place to investigate.

"...kids who drink raw milk are 41% less likely to suffer from asthma and allergies."
Journal of Allergy and Clinical Immunology, online
August 29, 2011

CHAPTER TEN

CHOICES

"Every person has free choice. Free to obey or disobey Natural Law. Your choice determines the consequence. Nobody ever did, or will, escape the consequences of his choices."
Alfred A. Montapert

Ultimately, the best diets consist of raw, organic, whole fruits, and vegetables. Add in some whole grains, legumes, and nuts. Red meat, pork, fish, and poultry should be free from antibiotics and growth hormones. These animals should be allowed to grow into maturity in a natural environment where they are exposed to fresh air, clean water, and sunshine. They should eat foods indigenous to their natural diets. These elements produce healthy animals and therefore healthy meat.

The best recommendation I can offer to improve our nutrition is to do our food shopping in a health food store or farmer's market and purchase organic products. Organic food is in a pure and unadulterated state, is more nutritionally dense, and is free from toxic pesticides and other industrial chemicals. The more man interferes in our food chain by violating natural law and over-processing our food, the more devitalized the food becomes.

Another obstacle to overcome when shopping organically is breaking old ingrained habits. I know that people have favorite brands of food and are resistant to change. Who wants to purchase natural peanut butter and deal with the oil separation when they can just as easily pick up a jar of hydrogenated peanut butter?

The organic products tend to be more expensive. With a family of five to feed, how many of us can afford these kinds of foods in bulk? Well, you can pay for health now or you can pay for sickness and disease later. Either way, you are going to pay. With money being the common denominator, the choice then becomes will you pay for health or will you pay for disease?

Have you checked the cost of disease lately? Open heart surgery runs the tune off some $15,000 plus hospital stay, doctor's visits, medications, and other associate care. Cancer treatment will run you hundreds of thousands. Even simple medications will leave your wallet begging for mercy. Ninety tablets of Lipitor (40mg) will run $135.00 or more. I'd rather invest a little more up front with organic products than have to face the bills that poor health can bring.

By keeping ourselves healthy we can be comfortable with larger insurance deductibles and co-pays. Ultimately, we can reduce our insurance premiums to cover only major medical expenses. As our body becomes more vitalized and healthy through better food choices, we will save money by not needing to see the doctor as much.

We can learn how to modulate our resistance to sickness through our foods. A broken bone will need medical attention. A cold will not. I am not demanding we become a card carrying member of the California Organic Alfalfa Sprouts Club overnight. I am, instead, stating that each step we take in the direction of better living can only reward us with better health. If we begin the journey hesitantly we will have hesitant results. Making small changes in our routine will affect a limited outcome.

If we cannot utilize a health food store or farmers market for whatever circumstance, we still can make better choices in the local supermarket. It is quite surprising to see just how easy it is to make better, healthier choices right where we shop. Many supermarkets are now carrying organic foods. So let's grab a shopping cart and get going!

Before we begin shopping, there are some basic ground rules we need to go over. We will not be aiming to reduce your choices but rather to read the labels and make better choices within the same product line. As we look down the aisles, our goal is to eliminate as much as possible the following non-food ingredients: processed sugars especially high fructose corn syrup, artificial sweeteners, hydrogenated fats, fried foods, all white colored foods including table salt, pasteurized milk, refined sugar, white rice, and bleached flour. Corn and soy products have all been contaminated with GMO (genetically modified organisms) so these should always be in organic form.

The white salt, sugar, rice, and flour have all been processed. Their nutritive factors have been bleached and stripped away. Years ago, when our grandparents stored real food in their pantries, there was a problem with keeping the bugs and mice from helping themselves to the wheat flour, brown rice and cane sugar. Because our grandparents used whole foods to prepare meals with, there was also a tendency for the foods to decompose if they were not used quickly.

Decomposition, rotting if you will, is a natural process of all organic matter. The food processing companies came up with the not so brilliant idea of stripping all the nutrition from the source and adding bleach just to make sure the destruction of all the nutrients was complete. They would then refortify these staples with some synthetic chemical versions of a few vitamins. This act of refortifying is equivalent to stealing a hundred dollar bill from our wallet and giving us back a quarter. Food processing insured that no bugs or mice would sneak into our pantry, for the bugs and mice are smart enough to know that this enriched, fortified non-food product has nothing to offer them in the form of sustenance. There is also much less chance of these white foods rotting now that the life essence has been denuded from them. What was once a complex food source, full of life giving qualities has been reduced to a nutritionally void product which is damaging to the digestive system. These bleached empty foods ferment in your digestive tract and upset the pH levels needed for proper digestion. This is just the beginning of a life time of malabsorption illnesses.

In most supermarkets, there is a complete aisle with nothing but soft drinks on one side and chips on the other. Neither of which can be considered "food" nor adds anything to our health quotient. The National Soft Drink Association stated that the consumption of soft drinks increased by 500% over the last 50 years. The average American drinks 275 milliliters of soft drinks per day which equals 26.5 gallons each year.[7] That number at first may seem implausible but when you consider the number of 36 to 64 ounce super servings that are purchased on a daily basis, it then does not seem so far-fetched. Do not forget the free refill offered at many fast food restaurants because we all know that the 32 ounces that comes with the meal is never enough. Is there a restaurant still left on the planet that serves an adult size soda that is smaller than 24 ounces? Since 1960, the soda industry has increased the single serving size from 6.5 ounces to 20 ounces.

Young males, ranging in age from 12-29 are the biggest consumers of soda at 570 milliliters per day which equates to 54.9 gallons per year.[8] Some of the sodas on the market today can contain as much as ten teaspoons of refined sugar in each can. That is enough sugar to raise your blood sugar levels to five times their normal range for four hours.

The high fructose corn syrup will be the hardest ingredient to eliminate from our new nutritional routine for it is used in almost everything. The danger in high fructose corn syrup is that it too has been devitalized

---

[7] A joint report from the American Dental Association and The Council on Scientific Affairs to the House of Delegates in October, 2001, in response to Resolution 73H-2000.
[8] Ibid

through processing and has been left with no semblance of nutrition. It has become a nutritional vacuum and as it passes through our body it will pull the minerals from our tissues to fill its own void.

This is basic physics involving equilibration. A condition of high volume will decrease when met with one of lower volume until the two become equal. Take two rooms separated by a door and heat one room to 90 degrees. When you open the door, the heat will move to the cooler room until the two rooms are the same temperature. High fructose corn syrup (or any other nutritionally void substance) steals the body's resources in the same manner. The high mineral content of the body is adsorbed into the corn syrup's void. These leached minerals are essential for proper function. Without chromium and zinc there is no insulin production. Boron helps stop bone loss. Iodine is needed for thyroid function. Deplete ourselves of magnesium and we may find our muscles become weak and our nerves become sluggish. We can ill afford (pun intended) to lose our minerals to high fructose corn syrup.

It is a mistake to think that we will be better off drinking diet sodas to avoid the sugar. The introduction of aspartame is yet another assault on the human biochemistry. It is a chemical compound that nature could never have put together herself. It is a molecule consisting of aspartic acid, phenylalanine, and methanol. Aspartic acid is a neurotoxin and can kill nerve cells. Phenylalanine is an amino acid needed for brain function. However, in the synthetic form and taken in excess without a balance of other amino acids, can lower serotonin levels and cause depression. The methanol is converted in the body into formaldehyde which is another neurotoxin and known carcinogen.

The chemicals found in soda can alter the pH of the body which has been implicated in many disease processes including arthritis. The phosphoric acid in the dark colored sodas can interfere with calcium absorption further complicating the condition.

Phosphorous needs to be in a certain ratio with calcium to be digested. If we overdose our system with sodas laden with phosphoric acid, our body will balance the load by pulling the needed calcium from our bones. Phosphoric acid has been shown to have the capability to erode the lining of our stomach. If we must drink soda we can all do ourselves a favor and switch to a natural soda. There are several companies to choose from. My personal favorite is R.W. Knudsen which uses sparkling water and concentrated fruit juice. Better yet, we can just drink clean water. After all, water is the *only* liquid essential to life.

It is no secret as to why the supermarket's entrances guide us to the fresh produce section of their store first. It is a sensory overload which enlivens our body. The colors, smells, and ability to touch the food stimulate our nervous system in a way that no can of beets or frozen corn could ever do. It puts us in good spirits to be around other living entities. Life begets life and the energies from the produce resonate with our own desires. (And try this experiment: Go into your local grocery store and stand in the produce section. How do you feel? Then try the same with a natural foods store brimming with organic produce. Can you "feel" the difference?) Load up the cart with anything you would like from here. We want to avoid irradiated and genetically engineered food. Remember, the more man tries to alter Mother Nature's perfection, the more trouble he puts himself in.

I do not need research from the very companies that sponsor this alteration of our food to tell me whether these options are of sound mind. If the Creator of Life wanted x-rays to interfere with biological processes our foods would be exposed to them naturally. If we were meant to have the genetic code of salmon in our tomatoes, they would already be there. Man does not need to meddle with that which is already in a state of perfection. Would you for one minute paint sunglasses on the Mona Lisa and declare it to be an improvement? Perfection is exactly that; Perfect. The circle of life has been in successful operation quite a bit longer than man's attempt to alter its natural course of action. Food is not a mistake that needs to be redesigned. How arrogant is man to believe he can improve on God's invention?

"Man's great desire is to pit 80 years against 80 million years; petty experiences against those aeons of time; perverted concepts to regulate worlds beyond his reach by reversing Natural Law to his artificial theories of how man can cure his physical or mental sickness and shortcomings."
B. J. Palmer

We can begin substituting our junk food snacks for fresh fruit and vegetables. When is the last time we sat back and tasted the tart refreshing snap of an apple? How long has it been since we crunched into the sweetness of a carrot? Remember as a child, squishing the banana through your teeth and showing the mashed up display to your siblings? Weren't celery stalks with peanut butter one of our favorite snacks? The coolness of a cucumber, the sharpness of a radish and the sour of the strawberries all wait to sacrifice their essence for us. Our mouth will come alive with a tropical luau when we eat pineapple, kiwi, and mango. Raisins, peppers, grapes, and melons are ready for our consumption. No boiling water, no frying pans, no preheated ovens; Just me and you and our precious, magnificent life once again remembering itself in the perfection of the life giving plum, orange, and broccoli.

As we shop, we will substitute our table salt with sea salt. Table salt is one of those processed white foods we want to eliminate. Unrefined Celtic sea salt contains all 84 minerals in precise doses that perfectly match the mineral makeup of your body. If we have a craving for salt, our body is really having a craving for not just sodium but also the other minerals that sodium chloride, table salt, does not provide. Our adrenal glands need sodium to function properly but it needs sodium in an unprocessed, mineral rich form. When our adrenal glands are faced with co-existing in an environment of mineral depleted sodium chloride, they will become weakened and we run the risk of experiencing a decrease in energy. Our adrenal glands are also responsible for regulating sexual development and function. Sodium deficient men can become less masculine and women can become less feminine.

For breakfast, maybe we would like some pancakes and maple syrup. If we reach for Hungry Jack Original pancake mix, we will experience a plate full of enriched bleached flour (enriched means synthetic vitamins have taken the place of the real vitamins, and there's some yummy bleach in there for us too), malted barley flour, sugar (there's too much processed sugar in our diets!), rice flour, baking powder, partially hydrogenated soybean oil (we are trying to stay away from hydrogenated oils), salt, calcium carbonate (an inorganic undigestible form of calcium) and nonfat milk. There is a box of pancake mix from Arrowhead Mills on the shelf. Let's see what they have to offer; organic buckwheat flour, organic whole grain wheat flour, organic soy milk powder, baking powder, and sea salt. All real foods, no chemicals. Get the idea?

Of course we plan on covering those pancakes with syrup. Mrs. Butterworth's Original Syrup will help us smother those pancakes with high fructose corn syrup, corn syrup (that's not a typo. We get corn syrup on top of corn syrup), water, salt, cellulose gum, molasses, potassium sorbate, sodium hexamethaphosphate (that sounds like a chemical to me,) citric acid, carmel color, (caramel color in colas and some other products is made by reacting sugars with ammonia and sulfites, two cancer causing toxins.) Be wary of the word artificial when used in any food product. Artificial means just that. It is not real. There is a glaring omission on this list of ingredients. Was there any mention of maple syrup? If we scan the label of Maple Grove Farms' maple syrup we will see some. In fact, 100% pure maple syrup with no preservatives is the only ingredient listed.

We will next pass right by the dairy cooler. I do not advocate pasteurized dairy products. My family gets raw milk, kefir, yogurt, cottage cheese, and butter from a local food co-op. If our state has made it illegal to sell raw milk in retail, we can check out www.realmilk.com to find a local outlet for raw dairy products (and farm fresh, free range chicken eggs.)

If we do buy store brand yogurt, don't just grab any old brand off the shelf. We must read the label. Just because we assume yogurt to be "health food" does not mean it is so. Yoplait's strawberry yogurt contains cultured, pasteurized, grade-A, low fat milk, and strawberries as we would expect. Look what else they have added; sugar, modified corn starch (beware of foods that have been modified), high fructose corn syrup, whey protein concentrate, kosher gelatin, citric acid, tricalcium phosphate, pectin, natural flavor, colored with carmine.

Compare that to the ingredients in Stoneyfield Farm's all organic yogurt: Cultured, pasteurized, organic low fat milk, naturally milled organic sugar, organic strawberries, inulin (fiber), pectin, annato extract (for color), natural flavor, and six live active cultures. Stoneyfield Farm's milk is free from bovine growth hormones. There are no artificial colors, flavors, sweeteners or preservatives. If those differences weren't enough to help you make a better choice, Stoneyfield Farm gives 10% of their profits to the efforts that help to protect and restore the earth.

How about some pasta for dinner? We will see the traditional brands of spaghetti list enriched (there's that word again) semolina, mononitrate, niacin, iron, thiamin, riboflavin, and folic acid. (Though they have vitamin names, they are synthetic chemical versions of the original whole vitamin complexes.) Hodgson Mill offers spaghetti made from 100% Duram whole grain wheat flour. Seems when a company uses a real food product, they do not need to enrich it with pseudo-wannabe-vitamins. They come prepackaged by Mother Nature in a whole, complete form.

We will need to purchase some sauce to top the spaghetti. Ragu Old World Style Traditional Sauce will give you a nice dose of tomatoes, extra virgin olive oil, salt, spices, Romano cheese, and dried onions, but then adds corn oil, high fructose corn syrup, and milk. Compare those ingredients to Safeway Select Garlic and Basil Pasta Sauce. Safeway Select uses tomatoes (puree, diced, paste), extra virgin olive oil, garlic, basil, salt, and spices.

Let's keep shopping. Kraft Boil in a Bag Minute Rice contains parboiled, enriched (enough said) rice, niacinamide, folate, ferric orthophosphate, and thiamine mononitrate. (Those words belong in a chemical test tube, not on our plate), Riceland Extra Long Grain Natural Brown Rice is made from exactly what the name says. That's it. No added chemicals and no fortifying or enriching.

Jiff Creamy Peanut Butter is made with roasted peanuts of course. Then they add sugar, partially and fully hydrogenated oils, molasses, mono and diglycerides, and salt. Saunder's Natural Creamy Peanut Butter is made from peanuts and salt. They add no trans fatty acids.

Let's compare more labels. Sunny D's recipe for quenching our thirst is comprised of water, high fructose corn syrup (it's everywhere, isn't it?), concentrated juices, citric acid, ascorbic acid, modified (food manipulation words pop up all over the place, don't they?) food starch, canola oil, sodium citrate, cellulose gum, xanthium gum, sodium hexamethaphosphate (that doesn't grow in your garden), sodium benzoate (a preservative), and yellow #5 and #6. Ever see an RDA for food coloring? Tropicana Pure Premium Orange Juice is made from oranges. No water, no preservatives and is sodium free.

Our choice for bread can be made with the same discretion. I recommend Ezekiel bread. The name comes from the Biblical reference. This recipe is thousands of years old and comes with God's stamp of approval.

"...take wheat, barley, beans, lentils, millet, and spelt, put them in one vessel and make them into bread for yourself."
Ezekiel 4:9

Ezekiel bread is made from the sprouts of unprocessed, real food and does not disrupt the digestive tract the way other nutritionally striped breads with gluten can. The sprouts provide more of a protein source instead of a carbohydrate one.

Potato chips can be exchanged for unbuttered organic popcorn. Eating more fish and less red meat will further address our desire for a healthier life. Here's another option we can ponder. Try a tablespoon of organic, unsulphured, blackstrap molasses in a cup of hot water instead of coffee. With very little imagination and just a tweak of our senses, we can taste a robust, coffee flavor with none of the jittery side effects. Plus, we receive the benefit of a good source of iron, potassium, calcium, magnesium, and an easily digestible form of sugar.

I can go on and on but I believe you are starting to understand that even in a traditional supermarket we can make better choices in our food selections. I am not asking that we make sacrifices. I am posing a challenge to think differently.

Every moment of our life is a direct result of the

choices only we can make. Right now, we are adults with the ability to change our mind. World peace is a choice. We have the choice to put down our weapons and shake hands or keep killing each other. I cannot be convinced that world politics is more complicated than that. It is not. In regards to your life, which do you choose: Health or disease? Do we choose fast food or a salad? Do we choose exercise or television? Do we choose soda or water? Do we choose natural medicine and body work or do we choose man made, toxic pharmaceuticals and surgery? We are the only ones who can determine the quality of our time spent on this planet. It is our choice.

> *"With every experience, you alone are painting your own canvas, thought by thought, choice by choice."*
> Oprah Winfrey

CHAPTER ELEVEN

LIFE VS. DEATH: NOT ALL SUPPLEMENTS ARE CREATED EQUAL

"One of the biggest tragedies of human civilization is the precedents of chemical therapy over nutrition. It's a substitution of artificial therapy over natural, of poisons over food, in which we are feeding people poisons trying to correct the reactions of starvation."
Royal Lee

If we are not eating at least six different raw fruits and vegetables each day, we need supplements. If we have ever been on a round of antibiotics, we need supplements. If we have ever suffered trauma, we need supplements. If we were not breast fed as a child, we need supplements. If we have ever passed soda or other processed sugar over our tongue or if we have ever eaten anything other than organic whole foods, we need supplements. If we have ever taken pharmaceuticals, we need supplements. If we have ever suffered an illness or are now confronted with a health concern, we need supplements. If we have children, pay taxes, or shop for the holidays, we need supplements. If we are exposed to any kind of man made stressor, such as those just listed, chemical, industrial, or agricultural pollution, we need supplements. If we are human and live on this planet, we need supplements. I think that just about covers it. Sounds a bit over the top doesn't it. I call it tough love. Read on.

First of all, we cannot get all our vitamins and minerals from the foods we eat today no matter what medical expert try to convince us otherwise. Next time a medical doctor tries to give advice on nutrition, ask them how many hours of nutritional training he/she received in medical school. The answer is surprising.

If our food comes in a box, can, bag, or carton it has been processed to some degree. Processing devitalizes an otherwise perfectly fortified food. Every time man touches food, the food becomes one more step removed from its natural state. Pasteurization, irradiation, genetic alteration, and chlorination all change the structural and functional makeup of the original food source. White bread is as far removed from its natural source as you can get. There is virtually nothing left in the white bread that resembles the wheat stalk from which it originated. By the time our favorite corn puff cereal reaches our bowl, there is no semblance of corn nutrition left. It is now just puffed air, synthetic pseudo-vitamins, and sugar. Rice does not grow snowy white and does not cook in a minute. Any kitchen that has witnessed this has not experienced rice as quality sustenance and neither has our belly. Processed food does not supply the same powerful nutritive value as real whole food. If we indulge in processed foods of any kind, we are cheating ourselves from the very nutrition our bodies crave.

Secondly, the soil from which our commercial foods are grown is depleted of minerals. Industrial farming has done a great job of abusing the soil. Where once family farms rotated crops to keep the cycle of the soil active, commercial farms plant the same crop over and over again. This does not allow for the soil to regenerate but rather continuously leeches the same minerals year after year. The farms are sprayed with synthetic chemical fertilizers, however, life begets life and you cannot regenerate life sustaining crops with synthetic man-made chemicals. Surely, crops grow from this environment but rest assured the crops are not replicas of Mother Nature's delicious design. The plants need more than just nitrogen and phosphorous to grow. There is a complete array of trace minerals essential for growth that is being ignored with synthetic fertilizers. The chemically treated crops are flawed with instructions foreign to the plants own needs for growth. Man-made chemicals, deficient in the complete needs of the crops, are not coded with life's genetic blueprint and therefore cannot create or enhance life. They are foreign, synthetic substances and no matter how remarkably close in design they are to the real thing, these artificial chemicals cannot replace God's design for life. This is a basic concept that is lost in the minds of science. Man can attempt to mimic life's processes in the laboratory but he will never succeed. Life, whether the conception of offspring, the balance of the food chain, or the process of evolution, all has its inspiration from a greater source. Man's involvement in recreating what is already naturally perfect will, in the end, create imperfection. This imperfection is filtered through man's limited senses and psychologically inspired bias. Science has draped a loin cloth over the statue of David and is trying desperately to pass it off as an improvement. If you eat food from an industrial farm, you need supplements.

Thirdly, man today is faced with more stress than ever before. Physical stress in the form of job security in an unstable world market, demands to work more for less pay, inflation, crowded highways and road rage all take their toll. Chemical stress via environmental pollution, all forms of drug use, and poor food choices decrease man's longevity. Emotional stress is a factor, whether it is manufactured from terrorism instilling fear, family structure decaying, trying to cope with ever increasing tax rates, or the breakdown in the ability to communicate. Common courtesies have been replaced with rudeness. Manners and respect have been pushed aside for poor behavior and a propensity for mischief. All of these factors wear down the body. The quality of the foods that we consume in today's age (unless you are 100% organic) does not equate to the level of stress posed upon our body. If we want to face the world and take on its challenges while being at our fullest potential, with all these stressors knocking at our door, we will need supplements.

So which supplements do we choose? In every genre of business there is good quality and there is poor quality. Just because the label says vitamin E or St. John's Wort does not necessarily mean that we will be getting a supplement that will have a beneficial effect to our physiology. Vitamins and supplements are as vastly different in quality as a Mercedes Benz and a Yugo.

Before I even get into a concentrated discussion of supplements, let's just take a quick look at some of the popular labels. If I am going to take a supplement, I want it to promote health. That seems like a reasonable request. I want to know what the ingredients are, what they do, and why they are in my supplement. Let's not even compare synthetic vitamins to a natural vitamin source, or which type of mineral is best absorbed just yet. For now, let's simply look down the list of ingredients of our bottle of multivitamins. Are there ingredients such as Sorbitol, Xylitol, Aspartame or sucrose? How about hydrogenated oil, FD&C Red # 40 or other colors? Does the label list artificial flavors, resin, starch, sodium benzoate as a preservative, or titanium dioxide? Is there a list of chemicals that only a scientist can pronounce? How do any of these ingredients promote health? They do not. They are fillers and additives used only to enhance the marketability of the product. If these companies were sincere in their desire to produce a quality product that enhances health rather than marketability, we would not have such ingredients in our vitamins. Processed sugars, artificial colors and preservatives are not food and therefore cannot feed our cells vital nutrition.

That simple and quick examination of our vitamins alone will eliminates most of the commercial brands of supplements as poor choices and may leave us scouring the health food stores for better options. Perhaps we were recommended a certain brand from our yoga instructor or our chiropractor sold us some from their office. The label may even read, "contains no wheat, dairy, gluten, artificial colors or preservatives" or even claim to be "all natural." Though that is certainly a step in the right direction, we can still make a better choice. There are always choices within choices.

The choice we are making here is the difference between whole food supplements and synthetic isolates. It is the difference between a supplement derived from a carrot and one fabricated from a man-made molecule called beta carotene. It is the difference between a supplement made from whole wheat germ sprung from Mother Earth and one manufactured in a sterile laboratory as d-alpha tocopherol. It is simply the difference between life and death. The two words here to key in on are synthetic and isolates. I want to address each word individually for they both have significant roles to play in decreasing the potency of our supplements.

Let's work with the isolates as a concept first. In September of 1992, the US Public Health Service recommended that all women in their child bearing years add 400 milligrams of folic acid to their diet. Science had discovered that adequate levels of folic acid help to prevent birth defects. Here is where I would question the research. Is folic acid the only B vitamin presented to us as a savior because the science community is agog with its own discovery? Why aren't the researchers raving about other B vitamins? Tell me, what are the benefits of thiamine, riboflavin, or biotin? Surely they can't be void of benefits just because science has not yanked the mystery from its molecular makeup. Look again at your multivitamin from your own cabinet. Do you notice how all the B vitamins are listed separately from each other? They are not listed as a complete complex but rather as fractionalized pieces of a once perfect whole. The truth is that no one B vitamin is more or less necessary at maintaining health than another. The B complex does not exist in nature as bits and pieces isolated from each other. There is no such thing as a thiamine flower or a niacin bush. There is a reason why it is called a complex.

To make matters worse, some nutrients are not acknowledged at all by the FDA as even being essential. Because research has not yet identified a magic bullet within certain elements, they have not been exalted to the level of acceptability. Who has ever heard of vitamin K? Vitamin K is needed to help the blood clot. It also aides in forming and repairing our bones. Vitamin K is essential in producing the protein in bone that crystallizes the calcium. It is one of the many factors responsible for the maintenance of a healthy liver as vitamin K converts glucose into glycogen.

How about vitamin B4? Vitamin B4, or choline in some circles, has been called an anti-paralysis vitamin. It promotes the proper function of nerves and can be utilized in conditions of irregular heart beat or fibrillations. It is utilized in the cell membrane to keep it strong and healthy. Vitamin B4 is good nutrition for the brain as it can improve mental function and memory. But alas, without the FDA stamp of approval, we are relegated to ignoring vitamins K and B4 as unimportant and useless elements.

Check the label of the multivitamin bottle once more. How is your vitamin C listed? Does your supplement say "as ascorbic acid"? Ascorbic acid is only one part of the entire vitamin C complex. Ascorbic acid is never found in nature without the rest of the vitamin C complex. The complete vitamin C complex is composed of a myriad of substances including bioflavinoids, flavinols, tyrosinase, P, K, and J factors, rutin, and hesperidin as well as an array of yet undiscovered elements. The ascorbic acid in our supplement is most assuredly a synthetic, isolated version of corn syrup. Whole foods are complete biologically active complexes that include enzymes, coenzymes, antioxidants, trace minerals, co-factors, and activators. This vast conglomerate of compounds works synergistically to create physiological changes in your body. They work together like no isolated fragment could ever do.

Ascorbic acid is the protective shell that binds all the other vitamin C components together. It is the Tupperware, if you will, that protects the rest of the molecules. Our body is smart enough to know that ascorbic acid does not occur in nature as a sole representative of vitamin C. When we consume isolated ascorbic acid, our body will question, in its own unique biological way, as to where the other parts of the vitamin C complex are. Ascorbic acid cannot be utilized properly by the body unless it is grouped with the entire vitamin C complex's cast of nutritives. Supplements made from whole food sources, rather than isolated fractions, supply all of nature's viable, necessary pieces; all of the discovered properties and, maybe even more importantly, all of the unknown, mysterious properties yet to be discovered.

In the same manner, d-alpha tocopherol is not vitamin E. Go ahead; check the bottle of vitamin E supplements on the shelf. If the label reads d-alpha tocopherol then you are getting an isolated fraction of the whole complex. Maybe the source lists vitamin E as mixed tocopherols. Well then, we are getting more than just the isolated d-alpha tocopherol aren't we? However, not only is vitamin E more than d-alpha tocopherol, it is more than mixed tocopherols. Vitamin E found in whole food sources contains four tocopherols, four tocotrienols, phospholipids, sex hormone precursors, selenium, the lipositols, and the xanthines. Ironically enough, each of these groups is a complex itself within the whole vitamin E complex. These groups work collectively as an antioxidant to support the immune system. They support cardiovascular health, improve circulation, and promote blood clotting. Vitamin E complex keeps the skin healthy, reduces scarring, and promotes healing. This team also works in concert with each other to support the reproductive system and its hormones. These functions of vitamin E are only what science has discovered thus far. Only God knows what magic is still hidden within the walls of the complete vitamin E complex.

Ascorbic acid is not vitamin C and d-alpha tocopherol is not vitamin E. They are isolates. They are pieces of a once vast network of perfection wrapped in divine mystery. Synthetic isolates are incomplete impostors. If our supplements lists its vitamins as fractionalized pieces instead of whole food sources we are wasting our money and may actually be causing deficiencies as our body continues to search every crack and crevice for real nutrition in a complete form. Vitamins in a natural state always exist as living complexes and never as isolated parts. It is the difference between a living entity and a dead chemical.

"No man is an island, entire of itself; every man is a piece of the continent."
John Donne

Science has done its best to reduce life to one individual, malleable unit. Their effort to dissect life into a strand of isolated DNA has certainly earned them historical notoriety. The entire concept of drug therapy is based on this reductionist thinking without consideration of the intact whole unit. One only has to listen to the advertisements on the television to understand this. Claritin may help you breathe easier but it is contraindicated in people who have hypertension, coronary artery disease, glaucoma, or urinary retention. Side effects include dry mouth, insomnia, headache, nervousness, fatigue and nausea. Prilosec is prescribed to treat the symptoms of acid reflux. Though the acid reflux may seem to be under control, one faces the possibility of diarrhea, flatulence, back pain, rash, and upper respiratory infection. This is isolated thinking for isolated parts that have gone bad without taking into consideration the effects on the whole structure.

Medical doctors will label a patient with high cholesterol as merely a high cholesterol problem. They may be prescribed Lipitor or Crestor to combat the elevated levels of cholesterol. However, cholesterol production is but one of the hundreds of functions of the liver. High cholesterol is, in part, a liver problem. All the blood in our body passes through the liver to be filtered. High cholesterol now becomes, in part, a toxic blood problem. The liver is intimately connected with the gallbladder which helps to process fats in the digestive tract. A dysfunction of fat metabolism contributes to high cholesterol. High cholesterol is, in part, a gall bladder problem. We cannot disturb one piece of the puzzle without upsetting the entire picture. Now, all of a sudden, high cholesterol is not just a cholesterol issue but involves the entire body as a malfunctioning whole. By treating just the cholesterol as an isolated issue, medicine is neglecting to focus on the Big Picture which is an imbalance of a greater magnitude within the body.

The entire ebb and flow of life, whether inside the human body or in the external environment, is interconnected in this manner. Ecological poisoning, oil spills, and hunting have managed to place the sea otter on the threatened species list. Sea otters feed on the sea urchin. The sea urchin consumes kelp from the ocean floor. As the otter's numbers decrease, the sea urchin populations increase. They, in turn, decimate the kelp beds, stripping them clean. The food chain has then been disrupted as there is no other animal to keep the sea urchin's numbers in check. The entire ecosystem of the kelp beds has been lost. Gone are the snails and other grazers that feed from the kelp. Gone are the fish that eat the grazers and use the kelp to hide themselves in. Gone are the sharks, orcas and sea lions that consume the smaller fish. Gone are the other bottom dwelling scavengers that feed from the scraps that land on the ocean's floor.

The sea otter is just one example of an infinite sampling of this synergistic role of nature. We cannot isolate one piece of a vitamin and ask it to act as the whole any more than you can separate the sea otter from the ocean and expect life to go on as normal.

> *"Synergy is the coordinated action of two or more agents so that the combined effect is greater than that of each part acting individually."*
> Mother Nature

Synergy is the effort of all parts working together to create a harmonious living condition. It is the very fabric of life. Without it, life ceases to exist. Isolated chemicals posing as whole vitamin complexes violates the very intent of eating God given food which is innately endowed with the complexity of synergism.

If the medical researchers today would look at a tree and examine it, they would dissect the tree to investigate its units individually. The scientist would comment on the leaves, bark, roots, and branches. A synergistic approach would distinguish itself from the traditional, analytical process by stressing the interactions of the tree with its surroundings. This would include how the tree cycles with the seasons, the life of the tree in relation to the whole forest, the habitat it provides for the animals and insects, describe the fruit and seeds the tree produces, the oxygen cycle, and the symbolism of the tree connecting the earth to the heavens. Interdependence is the glue that binds all life. The synergistic paradigm concentrates on the principles of organization. It focuses on the living system as a whole rather than cutting it into separate, individual pieces.

This exact concept of the whole being greater than the sum of its parts was reflected in a study done at the University of Illinois in which 32 patients with prostate cancer were asked to consume one tomato product (sauce, paste, fruit) each day for three weeks. Tomatoes have an important anticancer chemical called lycopene. In 2002, the results were published in *Experimental Biology and Medicine* in an article titled "Tomato Sauce Supplementation and prostate Cancer. It was noted that DNA damage from cancer had decreased 28%. The study concluded that there was a *"statistically significant result with the whole food regimen rather than isolated licopene."*

We can liken lycopene or any of these other isolated parts to a quarterback of a football team. We understand the importance of each in their respective areas. It can certainly be argued that the quarterback is the most important player on the team. He can pick which play to execute. He directs his teammates into position. He moves the offense down the field with accurate passing or precision hand offs. The games are won and lost depending on his performance. Likewise, lycopene has been identified as one of the most powerful anticancer elements known. There is much research defending lycopene's amazing power not only in fighting cancer but in reversing heart disease and age related macular degeneration. But to insinuate that the quarterback is the only player on the team would be ludicrous. In the same manner, lycopene is not the only beneficial quality in the tomato. The quarterback has the help of his coach, his front linemen, and his running backs and receivers. Even the roar of the home town fans bellowing down from the stadium seats will factor into the winning equation. The lycopene in tomatoes has the help of other phytochemicals, bioflavinoids, trace minerals, vitamins, enzymes, co-enzymes, and nutrients. By working in a synergistic manner, the quarterback and the lycopene become more efficient at performing their duties.

What this also implies is that the RDA's

established for each fractionalized, synthetic vitamin are not applicable when referring to whole food supplements. The RDA's are based on research done on each individual element. How much ascorbic acid (posing as vitamin C) is needed to prevent gum disease, or how much vitamin D is needed to prevent rickets, or how much calcium does one need to ward off osteoporosis may very well be titles of research programs but they fail to take into consideration the Big Picture. Though these kinds of studies may establish daily values for vitamins and minerals, they do not incorporate the synergistic actions of all the complimentary nutritives and co-factors. Vitamin E's RDA was established by testing synthetic alpha-tocopherol as a sole element. The studies do not examine the results of consuming wheat germ which is a whole food source of vitamin E complete with folic acid, magnesium, pantothenic acid, phosphorous, thiamine, zinc, co-enzyme Q-10, and PABA.

Remember, quantity is not synonymous with quality. Huge piles of imitation pieces do not equate potency. Do not be seduced by the "bigger is better" mentality. Ten milligrams of whole food supplement vitamin C complex will do our body more good than 1000 milligrams of synthetic ascorbic acid. What is needed is a balanced intake of the right whole food products for essential health and longevity. With respect to our food choices and nutrition, the whole is absolutely greater than the sum of its parts.

A whole food supplement has the advantage of utilizing the combined efforts of all the bound elements thus creating a more effective, efficient supplement. By utilizing a whole food supplement, one does not need the mega dosed daily values derived from synthetic isolate research. Milligrams do not measure potency. It measures weight. Quantity does not equate quality. We cannot extrapolate synthetically derived RDA's into whole food nutritive values. To do so would be akin to comparing apples to oranges. Of course apples and oranges are both whole foods so a more literal description would be to compare oranges to...well...ascorbic acid. What else? Synergy is the very fabric that binds life together. It is part of Universal Law. Nothing in our world can exist by itself without the cooperation of surrounding elements. Breathing is not just inhaling oxygen, health is not just the quality of your immune system, the spotted owl is not just another animal, a relationship is not just a passing hello, and vitamin C is not just ascorbic acid. The next chapter will discuss the dangers of the synthetic half of the phrase "isolated synthetic."

"Whole foods...have many benefits you can't find in a bottle. They're a complex package that provides many essential nutrients not just the few you may choose to take in supplement form. Whole foods contain hundreds to thousands of other substances...that may be important for good health. In fact, some food components may actually be detrimental to your health when taken as an isolated substance, such as in a supplement."
Mayo Clinic Health Letter, August, 1998.

CHAPTER TWELVE

SYNTHETIC VITAMINS ARE NOT VITAMINS AT ALL

synthetic > adjective 1. Made by chemical synthesis especially to imitate a natural product.

If our supplement is not from a whole food source then it is a synthetic replica. It has to be one or the other. Synthetically produced vitamins are a man made attempt to recreate nature. It is a nutritional fraud and can precipitate conditions worse than the original deficiency for which we sought to remedy. A synthetic vitamin is a counterfeit nutritional hoax. These fake attempts to mimic nature are at best drugs and can only have drug like effects on the body. At worst, they leave the body with greater deficiencies than when we began our supplemental protocol. A synthetic vitamin acts no differently than a drug. They are both chemical versions of a natural source and both produce reactions in the body that alter natural chemistry. Neither one addresses the vitality of the body as neither one of them has any nutritive factors that are essential to life. The atoms that make up synthetic vitamins are in a different configuration to their natural original design. The synthetic molecules can have some similarities to their natural counterpart but are in no way carbon copies. (Organic chemistry pun intended.)

This "close enough" mentality is why these counterfeit molecules are allowed to pass into our stores as vitamins. However, it is not the similarity of the molecules but the difference between them that cause debate. Thiamine hydrochloride and thiamine mononitrate are allowed to pass as thiamine in a vitamin but are completely different in their molecular structures. Any good chemist who has even the slightest inkling of quantum physics will tell you that any variation in a "look-a-like" molecule will have a profoundly different effect when it interacts with molecules in the body. The synthetic makeup of thiamine hydrochloride (or any other synthetic vitamin) is never found in any food matrix. It has never been part of our natural world it and never will be. Nature does not manufacture thiamine hydrochloride or thiamine mononitrate, therefore nature does not acknowledge or accept it as part of the system of life. Synthetic vitamins are not living foods. They are inert, dead chemicals. They are lifeless molecules.

The cells in our body have receptors along their outer membrane. For your vitamin, or any other element for that matter, to supply nutrition or information to the cell it must fit exactly inside the receptor. A lock and a key is a good way to describe this cellular coupling. Trying to squeeze thiamine hydrochloride into a thiamine receptor does not allow the cell to utilize the nutrition in a beneficial manner. This is akin to plugging your American hair dryer into a European electrical socket. The two systems are not compatible and the resulting connection has the potential to cause chaos. Not only does this improper receptor coupling not allow the cell to prosper but it also prevents other natural molecules from actually connecting to the cell. When our body is saturated with synthetic thiamine found in all the processed white flour products, real, natural thiamine, when you eat some, cannot attach to the cells. The receptors are full. By blocking the receptors, synthetic vitamins leaves the body just as depleted as it was before any vitamin was consumed. In its wake, it leaves behind toxic byproducts of the man made chemical synthesis which our body now has to work even harder to get rid of.

The *New England Journal of Medicine* published research in November 23, 1995 linking Vitamin A supplements to birth defects. However, only synthetic forms of vitamin A were used in the study. The research was careful to point out that vitamin A in the amounts and forms in actual foods did not result in birth defects.

While the high doses of synthetic vitamin A were shown to cause cleft lip and palette, heart malformations, and nervous system damage, real whole food vitamin A sources took the rap. Naturally occurring vitamin A was not found to be detrimental to the developing fetus. The fact is that the vitamin A in foods is essential to the development of the baby. Naturally occurring vitamin A is needed for all cell differentiation and organ development especially in the eyes and bones.

Another citing from the *New England Journal of Medicine*, April 14, 1994, noted similar finding with smokers and the effects of consuming beta-carotene and vitamin E. Science again utilized man made forms of these vitamins and found the results to be quite contrary to the belief that these two vitamins could help protect us from the ravages of cancer. The synthetic vitamin E produced more strokes while the synthetic beta-carotene showed an 18% higher incidence of lung cancer. This counterfeit form of nutrition fails time and time again to produce a healthy outcome. Synthetic, manmade vitamins are not vitamins at all. They are a poor attempt to duplicate nature's actions. We cannot fit a left hand into a right handed glove comfortably any more than you can expect synthetic thiamine hydrochloride to fit into a natural thiamine receptor.

This information is by no means new to the scientific community as seen by this finding published in Annual Review of Biochemistry, 1943:

"Natural forms of vitamin E lose up to 99% of their potency when separated from their natural synergists."

Since industries started manipulating our food supply so it would fit inside a box and sit on a grocery shelf for months at a time, voices have been raised to caution us against this destructive practice. As far back as the mid to late 1930s, nutritional pioneers Royal Lee, Weston Price, Francis Pottenger, Melvin

Page, and John Tilden were leading the battle to educate the people on the deteriorating health conditions caused by processed food.

Again, it is not my attempt to cite reference after reference and bore you to death with research. Suffice to say that there exists a mountain of literature, citations, and clinical evidence supporting the principles that whole foods function as biological life sustaining complexes while synthetically designed nutrients fail to do the same. Most of this information was gathered in a time before special interests and political advantage worked their way into the outcomes of the research.

Once these corrupting influences secured themselves into the mix, right and wrong no longer became the driving impetus to the truth. False assumptions and flawed theories penetrated the mainstream ideas and supported personal greed and power instead of the facts. Once people were brainwashed into believing that fortifying nutritionally stripped foods with synthetic vitamins was a sound practice, then no connection to nutritionally related disease could possibly exist. The mindset became something to the effect of, "if we are receiving our daily dose of vitamins via fortified or enriched white bread, rice products, or breakfast cereals, how can we possibly have any nutritional deficiency?" For the last 60 years or more science has turned its back on the relationship of degenerative disease and nutrition believing in the absurdity of replacing whole food nutrition with chemical frauds.

Doctor Royal Lee, founder of Standard Process, a whole food supplement company, was a pioneer in the nutritional industry. He, along with just a handful of other nutritional proponents, took on the food processing industry in the early to mid 1940's. They tried in earnest to reveal the flawed ideals of synthetic vitamins to the public. When push came to shove however, and the food processing companies began to feel the heat from the realization that the truth concerning the dangers of synthetic vitamins was being exposed, Dr. Lee felt the full weight of the political influence of these special interest groups. He was eventually ordered by the courts to burn his research papers which supported his points of view and a gag order was issued. So much for freedom of speech. Long live our Bill of Rights.

The irony here is quite obvious. In a time when medical doctors were advertising cigarettes as a digestive aid and soft drinks were touted to keep our appetite under control, Dr. Lee's information was being suppressed. Even today the Constitution allows people such as Larry Flint and his Hustler magazine to flourish under the freedom of speech amendment while others must bight their tongues. Pedophiles under the guise of NAMBLA can propagate their perversion upon our land but we are not allowed to hear of the health benefits of certain vitamins and herbs. The medical researchers, lost in their own ego based ignorance, are acting like ostriches with their heads stuck in the dirt. If the body does not know the difference between artificial vitamins and natural, whole food sources of vitamins, why are we able to recover artificial vitamins in the urine and undigested vitamin pills in the septic waste?

There are a few other whole food nutritional companies available to us and we certainly have the freedom to explore them all and find the one that best suits each one of us. Be careful of sales gimmicks. Some hold merit. Some do not. For example, companies that promote whole food supplements in liquid form will tell you they have studies proving liquids digest and absorb better than tablets. We should find out if those studies were done while comparing the liquid supplement to synthetic vitamins or other whole food supplements. A whole food supplement in solid form will digest just as well as any liquid. Our nourishment mostly comes in solid form, doesn't it? It turns into a liquid through the process of digestion all on its own. That's how nature designed it to be. Digestion takes care of the rest. The liquid debate does not then hold merit.

For all the reasons cited above, I recommend Standard Process whole food supplements to all those who wish to supplement their nutritional needs. This philosophy of nourishing the body with whole foods is reflected in their products. I have been using Standard Process in my office for many years and I have witnessed the success stories first hand. Healing is found in the wholeness of nature's abundance not in the test tube of a chemist.

"Drugs never cured disease. They merely hush the voice of nature's protest and pull down the danger signals she erects."
Daniel Kress

CHAPTER THIRTEEN

ADD SOME PUNCH TO YOUR LUNCH (or any other meal)

"The art of medicine consists of amusing the patient while nature cures the disease."
Francois Voltaire

Most people become overwhelmed when confronted with changing poor lifestyle choices. This is because they have been given a list of dos and don'ts a mile long and they are expected to change all of their bad habits overnight. Ideally, that would be great but let's first start out with some more practical ideas. We have to crawl before we can walk so taking it slow may provide a better transition for us. I'm suggesting that we start by choosing better alternatives. Here are some of my favorite, quick, simple additions we can make to our daily or weekly routine without concerted travail. They each, in their own way, provide powerful nutrition with minimal effort. By adding these suggestions to our regimen, we can begin to regain a quality of life that we deserve. These are not sacrifices but rather compliments. With very little effort, we can immediately begin to reap the benefits of some of the most powerful, healthy foods on earth. Please remember that the best results will come from using organic sources that have not been processed. Stay away from products that have been filtered, heated, and refined.

1. **Fruit Smoothies**. This is a great breakfast for those on the go. Instead of grabbing a donut or toaster pastry and running out the door, try this idea. Fill a blender with a cup or two each of several different fruits. Some enjoyable combinations are pineapple, banana, strawberry, or apple, pear, cinnamon. We can combine several different berries; blueberry, raspberry,

strawberry and create a delicious drink. Mango, kiwi, and pineapple combine for a tropical flavor. There is an infinite combination of smoothies available to us if we use our imagination.

I also put half an avocado in the mix. The avocado has a simple flavor that blends completely with the fruit. It is a superfood loaded with fiber, vitamins K, C, B6, E, folate, niacin, pantothenic acid, potassium, copper, manganese, and magnesium. It also has the good fats our body needs. Add a couple of spoonfuls of plain yogurt or kefir (best in a raw dairy form from a local food co-op) for some probiotics and a farm fresh egg.

Yes, I said an egg. After we blend the mixture together, we will never taste the egg but we will feel the health benefits of a raw protein source, zinc, sulfur, lecithin and more. Nor am I concerned with salmonella. Farm fresh eggs from pasture raised organic chickens are not to be feared. Healthy chickens lay healthy eggs. Eggshells are porous. When an egg is laid, it is covered with a protective coating call the "bloom" that seals the pores in the eggs. This prevents bacteria and other pathogens from entering the egg.

Industrial farm eggs are washed in hot water mixed with detergent, chlorine and/or ammonia. With the bloom washed off, the chlorine and ammonia can seep into the egg. Next time you sit down to a breakfast of eggs and bacon, ask yourself, "What's the RDA for chlorine or ammonia?"

Before the eggs head off to the store they are finally covered with a thin film of clear, odorless oil. This is to artificially replace the bloom and protect the egg. Eggs produced in factory farms have a higher rate of food poisoning due to bacteria from the unhealthy way chickens are raised and eggs are treated. (More on the egg later.)

The yogurt or kefir provides the active cultures that will aid in the health of the digestive system. Our fruit gives us live enzymes so desperately needed in today's world of cooked food and we are rewarded with a multitude of vitamins and minerals from the assorted fruit.

To add even more nutrition and health insurance to the mixture, I recommend Standard Process's SP Complete. SP Complete is a vegetarian whole food powder supplement which provides the body with essential vitamins and minerals. It contains whey protein, flax meal, brown rice protein, buckwheat, barley grass, and twenty one other whole foods and botanicals.

We can pour this concoction into our favorite 32 ounce big gulp cup and off we go to work. By sipping this through the morning hours we will be providing ourselves with more nutrition than most people see in several days.

2. **Ginger Root Tea**. The medicinal properties of ginger are older than recorded time. Ginger is most noted as a digestive aid helping minimize the symptoms of morning sickness, motion sickness, and chemotherapy related nausea. It can also help heal ulcers. Ginger has antiseptic properties and aids in keeping the inside of the body clean from unwanted bacteria, virus, and fungus. It promotes cardiovascular health by stimulating circulation, decreasing cholesterol, and decreasing blood clots. It also has anti-cancer properties and can ease the discomfort of inflammation especially that associated with arthritis. Ginger can boost your energy level. Ginger is common enough so that you can purchase it from most any grocery store. Cut off a piece about one inch long. Slice this chunk into thin pieces. This can make about two cups of tea depending on one's taste. Drop the ginger root into a pot of water and bring it to a boil. Once the water reaches a rolling boil, turn down the heat and let it simmer for about fifteen minutes. Strain off the chunks of ginger and presto; we have a mug full of healing wisdom. Add honey or lemon to taste or just sip it as is. We can make extra ahead of time and keep it in the refrigerator. It makes a great cool beverage as well.

3. **Raw Honey.** Raw unpasteurized honey is mankind's oldest sweetener. It promotes energy as it is a rich source of complex carbohydrates and protein. Honey is a source of Vitamins B, C, D, and E. Raw honey can be used to help eliminate allergies to pollen. Its antibacterial properties help in wound healing including ulcers. Honey's antioxidant properties can help in the prevention of cancer. A topical application of honey can make a salve beneficial in wound healing, burns, bed sores, and cuts. Children under one year of age should never eat honey. Their digestive tracts are not mature enough to process the honey correctly and the spores in the honey can cause botulism. This is of no concern to the mature digestive tract however so eat up. A spoonful is all it takes to add this amazing nectar to our daily diet. If the taste is too sweet we can use a spoonful in our ginger root tea or spread it out on a piece of toast made from Eziekial bread. Stir a spoonful into some yogurt or cottage cheese. There is more nutrition and health benefits in a spoonful of raw unpasteurized honey than in any fast food meal deal on the planet.

4. **Flaxseed**. Flaxseed is another ancient medicine which has been severely ignored in today's diets. I can only imagine how much healthier the people of this country would be if our bread was made from, or at least had some flaxseed in it. The flaxseed is loaded with omega-3 fatty acids and lignans. These two elements, combined with the other properties of flaxseed, can improve cardiovascular health by decreasing cholesterol, and prevent strokes and heart attacks by thinning out blood clots. It can ease the symptoms of menopause. Flaxseed has anti-inflammatory properties which help those who suffer from arthritis. It contains B vitamins, protein and zinc and is a great fiber source that will eliminated constipation. Flaxseed has shown to have antibacterial, antifungal, antiviral, and anticancer properties. Flax in its whole seed source is the least processed of all the flax oil sources. Crunching a spoonful a day will aid in your journey into acquiring

better health. Once the seed has been ground, the nutritional qualities become very fragile. Light and air can destroy much of the ground flaxseed's healing properties. Grinding flaxseed and using it immediately is the best way to enjoy its health benefits. If we choose a ground source of flaxseed, make sure it is packaged in a dark container that keeps out the light. Keep it in the refrigerator and keep the package tightly closed. We can, like the honey, just eat a spoonful by itself, or we can mix the flaxseed into our yogurt, cereal, or cottage cheese.

5. **Apple Cider Vinegar.** Apple cider vinegar was revered by the great cultures of Egypt, Greece, and within the Roman Empire. This miraculous tonic has been touted as one of the world's most powerful medicines. Look in any nutritional reference and you will see an endless list of maladies that can be helped by adding apple cider vinegar to one's diet. It promotes digestion by helping to breakdown stagnant food in the stomach. Acid indigestion or reflux is a misnomer. Most stomach complaints are not due to too much stomach acid but rather too little. The food in our stomach cannot be broken down effectively because of a lack of acid production. The rotting food gives off putrid gasses much like a compost pile. It is these gasses that can give the feeling of burning in the esophagus. The reflux of stomach acid is more conjecture than fact. By drinking two teaspoons of organic apple cider vinegar (diluted in a small glass of water) after a meal, we will notice the symptoms of indigestion soon become a thing of the past.

Apple cider vinegar is noted as an arthritic medicine as it is able to break down calcium deposits in the joints while mineralizing the bones. It helps to balance the blood pH levels which are critical in maintaining any degree of optimal health. Apple cider vinegar is an antiseptic as it is a noted germ killer.

I personally drink apple cider vinegar with my

evening meal. I put two tablespoons in a glass of water (not from the tap) and add a tablespoon of raw honey. The raw honey takes the twang out of the vinegar and the vinegar takes the sweet out of the honey. With this combination we have successfully consumed two foods from this list at once. This is a delicious, refreshing drink that will have you craving more. The only apple cider vinegar I use is Bragg's apple cider vinegar as it is raw, unfiltered, and unpasteurized. Nutritional status and enzymes are destroyed with pasteurization. Please check out their website at www.bragg.com

6. **Garlic.** Garlic's potent medicinal qualities have been used for over 5,000 years. It is one of the most viable foods on the planet. It has an endless array of benefits. Garlic can help lower blood pressure, cholesterol, and decrease the incidence of blood clots. Garlic is a natural antibiotic and was used in World War I to treat infections and gangrene. Its high selenium content is a potent immune stimulant. It is effective in fighting fungal infections including Candida, athlete's foot, and vaginitis. Garlic keeps the blood and the body clean from unwanted germs and bugs. Garlic has been shown to have the ability to kill parasites and cancer cells. The oil in garlic is beneficial to the heart, colon, and is effective in treating arthritis and circulation problems. What more could we want in a food?

A garlic press is an easy way to mince a clove and add the magic to our foods. Garlic can be added to all our meals that include pasta sauce. Add a clove or two to a stick of melted butter and create your own garlic butter. You can even refrigerate the unused portion Add it to your mashed potatoes or other vegetables. Chewing on a sprig of parsley after garlic can help to refresh the mouth.

7. **Cold Pressed Extra Virgin Olive Oil.** This powerful gem is the secret behind the popular Mediterranean

diet. It is a powerful antioxidant and can help slow down the appearance of aging. It keeps the muscles and skin soft and subtle. Olive oil protects against colon, breast, and skin cancer. Mediterranean cultures are famous for their sunny coastlines and warm vacation destinations yet they have a low incidence of skin cancer. Olive oil can lower cholesterol and blood pressure. It can relieve constipation and aid in digestion. Olive oil has also been shown to help heal coronary heart disease and arteriosclerosis.

How quick and easy would it be for us to take our bottle of olive oil out of the cupboard and swallow a tablespoon. Talk about giant gain with minimal effort. Doing this each day will surely promote a healthier state. Extra virgin olive oil has a simple, soft taste that is quite palatable. There should be no need to run from this recommendation with a sour face.

8. **Yogurt.** The history of fermenting foods predates written time. The fermenting of milk into yogurt changes the entire dynamic of the milk. Yogurt promotes healthy digestion. The live cultures found in the yogurt have changed the lactose (milk sugar) into lactic acid. Calcium needs an acidic environment to be absorbed and the lactic acid provides just that. The yogurt also enhances the absorption of other nutrients as well. It enhances the immune system by overpowering E. Coli, Salmonella, Staphylococcus, Listeria and Candida. For this reason, yogurt helps to decrease the incidence of bladder and vaginal infections.

Helping ourselves to some yogurt three times a week (or daily for best results) will provide us with this added defense against disease. Yogurt is a small snack with a big payout. Here is an important note. Just because the cup on the store's shelf says yogurt does not mean it is health food. There are lots of brands of yogurt out there that are filled with nonfood stuff. I highly recommend farm fresh yogurt but if you choose a store bought brand, the brand that I recommend for its organic purity and attention to quality is Stonyfield. Compare labels and see for yourself.

9. **Eggs.** This little, often maligned food is not only inexpensive but very versatile. Best of all, it is loaded with nutrition. It is one of the best protein sources available. The egg (farm fresh complete with mud, dirt, small feathers, and chicken poop stuck to the shell) supplies choline which is good for the nerves and brain. Choline helps prevent fat build up in the liver. Our egg will supply us with nearly every vitamin and mineral we need including vitamin A, the B vitamins of folic acid, niacin, riboflavin, and B6. The egg also provides magnesium, zinc, and iron. These are essential minerals needed for energy production, calcium absorption, prostate gland function, immune system vitality, and the oxygenation of red blood cells.) Don't fall victim to the cholesterol scare tactics. The cholesterol in eggs is a natural source used to make vital steroids and sex hormones. The egg contains lecithin which is a natural fat emulsifier. It will break down the cholesterol and make it available for the cells to use. Raw eggs are better than cooked so add one to your smoothie today!

Here is the all important question. How many of us have these items in our pantries, refrigerators, or kitchens right now? Reread the health benefits for each of these select foods and compare them to the major diseases of today. This is one of the key factors why so many Americans have succumbed to degenerative disease at such young ages and at such alarming rates. People have traded these miracles of life for potato chips, aspartame, sugared cereal, fast food, high fructose corn syrup, and cookies. We have forgone the benefits of vinegar, garlic, ginger, fruits, vegetables, honey, olive oil, yogurt, and flaxseed for processed, bleached flour, canned vegetables, candy bars, designer coffee, and hydrogenated fat. By adding these essential super foods to our own diet, we can ward off high cholesterol, high blood pressure, arthritis, heart disease, diabetes, cancer, digestive problems, and so much more. The foods I have listed above take so very little effort to incorporate into our routine that there is really no excuse not to. The payback in terms of health benefits is infinite. We cannot get that kind of protection from what has become the staple of the American fast food diet.

There certainly are many other wonderful, powerful, nutritious foods that can be added to our regimen. Ginseng, kelp, broccoli, oat bran, spirulina, wheat germ, kale, and bee pollen deserve honorable mention. The shitaki, reishi, and maitake mushrooms also have superior healing and detoxifying qualities. Any piece of fresh fruit or a salad brimming with vegetables is always a good nutritional choice. It is not my intention to single out any one food over another. The idea is to begin to add real food back into our diet and eliminate the processed, refined, synthetically fortified, non-nutritive fillers.

We must also note the difference between a meal and a snack. The size of our portions has as much to do with our health as does the quality of the food itself. If we eat ice cream (Breyers is all natural and organic is even better) one scoop is a snack. Three scoops are ridiculous. If we stop at a sandwich shop for lunch, a six inch sandwich is adequate. A twelve or sixteen inch sandwich is gluttony. Stuffing our stomachs full at each meal puts undue stress into the digestive system. Excess stress will cause premature damage to any system whether it is anatomical or mechanical.

"Our body is a machine for living. It is organized for that, and it is its nature. Let life go on in it unhindered and let it defend itself, it will do more than if you paralyze it by encumbering it with remedies."
Leo Tolstoy

CHAPTER FOURTEEN

DRINK UP!

"Water is H_2O, hydrogen two parts, oxygen one, but there is also a third thing that makes water and nobody knows what that is."
D. H. Lawrence

One of the most important pieces of advice in regards to improving your health and the easiest to accomplish would be to drink more of clean, pure water. My patients look at me like I am from Mars when I suggest that drinking more water can help them reduce their back pain or attain a healthier overall disposition. It is the *only* fluid our body demands we partake of. When we feel thirsty, the only drink we need to quench that sensation is water.

All wild animals, as well as most of our pets drink nothing but water. Humans are animals too so why would the rules of nature be any different for us? All other animals can survive without soda, beer, and coffee and so can we. What happens to our house plants or our vegetable garden if they do not receive enough water? They shrivel up and die. Our body does the same thing. If the only thing we ever drank from this day forward was clean, fresh water, we would be a healthier person for it.

Hardly anyone drinks enough water. Most people walk around in a perpetual state of dehydration. Coffee, alcohol, and soda have become co-conspirators in an attempt to further deplete the hydration of the body. The body is made up of 70-80% water. Therefore, one would assume that to maintain the integrity of the human body we must keep that percentage intact. As our body uses water every day, it must be replaced.

There are many formulas to determine how much water one should drink in a day. One rule of thumb is to drink 6-8 glasses of water daily. However, I find this piece of advice falls short. This does not take into consideration your body size or your activity level. Children can not drink as much water as adults. People who work in manual labor, especially in the hot sun, require more water than the rest of us. Another calculation recommends that we divide our body weight in half and that is how many ounces of water we should drink in a day. A 150 pound person should consume 75 ounces of water or about nine, eight ounce glasses.

As a young bachelor, I asked my grandmother one day, "How long do you cook a chicken for?" Her reply was, "Until it's done." This seems like reasonable advice when it comes to the water issue. Drink until we are done. Carry a bottle with us everywhere we go and sip from it all day. Keep it on our desk at work. Carry it to the car. By sipping water all day we will be surprised at just how easy it is to drink a liter or more of water.

I am not a proponent of drinking water with meals as the water dilutes the stomach acid. If we do drink water with meals, make sure our drink is mixed with Bragg's apple cider vinegar and raw unpasteurized honey. These add great digestive enzymes to our meal. At breakfast, ginger tea (hot or cold) has not only added more water to our regimen but has also added some powerful healing medicine as well. An added benefit from increasing the amount of water we drink is that it will decrease the amount of non-water drinks we consume. Every glass of water that we drink means one less glass of soda or coffee.

Sipping in lieu of gulping also prevents frequent trips to the bathroom. The sips of water are used by the body continuously. Chugging full glasses of water just to meet our drinking quota will quickly overload the digestive and urinary systems causing us to visit the bathroom more often. Do not set unrealistic goals as to how much one should drink. Remember, drinking some water is better than not drinking any at all. If the taste of water is too boring and we need more flavor on our tongue, try a squeeze of lemon or lime. Once again, we are adding great nutrition as well as flavor to the water. How many days has it been since you last drank fresh, clean water?

    Water is essential to all our bodily functions. Every cell in our body is dependent upon water. It would be a laborious task to list all the benefits of drinking water but here are some of the obvious ones. Water helps to regulate our internal temperature controls. It filters toxins and removes waste products. It carries nutrition and oxygen to our cells. Water is essential to proper digestion and absorption of food. We need water to lubricate our joints and cushion our internal organs. It is required to balance the pH factors of our different body parts. Water helps to rid the body of fat. It is integral in maintaining blood pressure.

    Water comprises 80% of our world and interestingly enough it makes up approximately 80% of our body. Understand this; whether we talk about 85% of our soft brain or 20% of our hard bones, our body is not made up of root beer, coffee, milk shakes, or any kind of high fructose corn syrup thirst quencher laced with synthetic vitamins and indigestible minerals. Our body is filled with water so drink up!

    Unfortunately, in most areas of this country, our tap water is not suitable for sustaining a healthy internal environment. Because of toxic run off from factories and farms, our water supply has become contaminated. We share our water supply with our sewers. Some potentially hazardous contaminants commonly found in tap water include benzene, arsenic, nitrates, and heavy metals such as lead, cadmium, and mercury. Asbestos, phosphates, carbon dioxide, pesticides, treated sewage, radioactive particles, pharmaceuticals, bacteria and viruses such as giardia and cryptosporidium can round out the ingredients in our glass of tap water. Kind of makes you want to chug down a big glassful right now doesn't it? What if we could add alum and polymers to settle out the dirt? Could caustic sodas, ferric chloride, and lye used to prevent pipe corrosion and soften water do the trick?

> *"Water and air, the two essential elements on which all life depends, have become global garbage cans."*
> Jacques Cousteau

Who could forget the inspirational story of Erin Brockovich as she exposed the world to the leaching of chromium 6 by the Pacific Gas and Electric Company into the water supply of Hinkley, California? I am sure that PG & E is not the only business in this country that has contaminated the ground water. The next Erin Brockovich movie could take place right in our own backyard.

The government adds even more poison to the water in the form of chlorine under the guise of improving the quality of the water by making it cleaner and therefore safer to drink. A proactive mind set would be one that protects the pristine water supply from becoming contaminated in the first place. It would force farms to find alternatives to toxic chemical pest controls and synthetic fertilizers. (Sounds like organic farming to me.) It would force industry to be liable for the pollution it creates. Instead we are once again faced with the stigma of covering up the symptoms (chlorinate the polluted water to kill the germs) versus addressing the cause of the problem itself (stop polluting the water). This is yet another example of becoming an "aspirinoholic".

The chlorine is meant to disinfect the water but it is a poison nonetheless. Webster's New Universal Unabridged Dictionary defined chlorine as a greenish-yellow, *poisonous*, gaseous chemical element with a *disagreeable odor*, used in the preparation of *bleaching agents*, in water purification, in various industrial processes, *as a lung irritant in chemical warfare*, etc. (italics added for emphasis.) Chlorine, its byproducts such as ammonia, and its compounds such as trihalomethanes are known carcinogens. Would we ever consider walking into our laundry room and taking a big swig of our bleach? Keep drinking tap water and that's exactly what we'll get. Chlorine is chlorine and even in minute doses it is a toxin to the body.

Fluoride is another water additive that is meant to be beneficial. The purpose of fluoridating our water was to help prevent tooth decay. Fluoridation safety studies are some 50+ years old. A quick history lesson can show us that fluoridation was found to be safe in an era when we were told that cigarette smoking was good for you and do not worry about DDT because it only killed bugs. A rose is a rose and a toxin is a toxin. Industrial fluoride is not a rose. That is for sure. It has been linked to thyroid disease, arthritis, brain damage, and cancer. Austria, Belgium, Denmark, Finland, France, Germany, Iceland, Italy, Luxembourg, Netherlands, Norway, Sweden, Switzerland, and most of the United Kingdom have reevaluated the use of fluoride due to its toxic makeup. There is a mountain of evidence today that suggests that fluoridated water is unnecessary and harmful.

According to the handbook, Clinical Toxicology of Commercial Products, fluoride is more poisonous than lead and just slightly less poisonous than arsenic. It is a cumulative poison that stores up in bone over the years. From 1990 to 1992, *The Journal of the American Medical Association,* published three separate articles linking increased hip fracture rates to fluoride in the water. In the March 22, 1990 issue of *The New England Journal of Medicine*, Mayo Clinic researchers reported that fluoride treatment of osteoporosis increased hip fracture rate and bone fragility.

Surprisingly, the most recent studies do not even show that water fluoridation is effective in reducing tooth decay. In the largest U.S. study of fluoridation and tooth decay, United States Public Health Service dental records of over 39,000 school children, ages 5-17, from 84 areas around the United States showed that the number of decayed, missing, and filled teeth per child was virtually the same in fluoridated and non-fluoridated areas.

Bottled water comes with its own list of dangers. These plastic containers have been implicated in leaching dangerous chemicals into the water they hold. DEHA (diethylhydroxylamine) is a known carcinogen and BPA (Bisphenol A) has been cited as causing neurological and behavioral problems. BPA is a xenoestrogen, a known endocrine disruptor. These synthetic xenoestrogens are linked to breast and uterine cancer, decreased testosterone levels in men, and are especially devastating to babies and young children.

I'm not a fan of these new "vitamin" waters that have flooded the market either. These products are loaded with sugar (crystalline fructose is a name used to disguise the word sugar) to which some synthetic vitamins have been added. A bottle of vitamin type water can contain 33 grams of sugar (one bottle of Vitamin Water is 2.5 servings x 13 grams/serving) making it more akin to a soft drink than to any semblance of a healthy beverage. Health experts concur that all these added sugars in our diets plays a key role in our obesity epidemic, a problem that now leads to more medical costs than smoking.

I want us to hydrate all day everyday with clean fresh water but I have warned about the dangers of using tap water, bottled water or any type of vitamin laden water. What are we to do? At my house, my family uses an under the sink filter from Wholly Water. The Wholly water filter will remove chlorine, lead, fluoride, mercury, barium, arsenic, trihalomethane, aluminum, radon, chromium, sulfur, iron, uranium, cadmium, pesticides, insecticides, fertilizers, benzene, PCBs and a truck load of chemicals I cannot pronounce. It is self cleaning with no cartridges, filters, or membranes to change. It eliminates contaminants but allows healthy minerals to remain.

Then, on top of the counter, we have a Kangen water machine connected to the faucet. The Kangen water machine has many, many special features. One of these features is creating alkaline ionized water. The standard American diet (soda, liquor, coffee, processed meats, fried food) can disrupt the precious pH balance in the body by creating an acidic environment. Cancerous tumors thrive in an acidic environment. Of course minding our diet and eating our green leafy vegetables is our first line of defense in disease but Kangen water allows for some great insurance.

The Kangen machine also creates water that is extremely high in antioxidants. The molecules also become micro-clustered which allows for instant absorption into the cells. I would caution against purchasing cheaper machines. Many fall short of their claims with limited technology and poor manufacturing. Without wanting to sound like a commercial sponsor, I will direct you to the website www.waterpollutionfilters.com. Here, you can read much more about these products.

Anytime man processes food (or water), the nutritional life sustaining quality diminishes. If our food and water does not come to us directly from the source (the Earth) it has been processed to some degree. The more processing, the less vital. If our food is precooked, enriched, canned, fortified, modified, hydrogenated, frozen, boxed, bagged, chemically or genetically altered, it is devitalized and most likely void of its original God given state of "aliveness". It is dead empty food. The same is true for water. Processing water stripes this vitality from the molecules much the same way as processing food denatures it.

The more our body stays hydrated and alkalinized with water high in antioxidants, the better health we will enjoy. The quality of our life will absolutely improve with every can of soda that we replace with fresh clean water. Soda is a man made drink and contributes nothing to our nutritional needs. Water is a God given, life sustaining drink that has everything to do with our biological functions. Without it we would not exist. With it we will live.

"We must pay respect to water, and feel love and gratitude, and receive vibrations with a positive attitude. Then, water changes, you change, and I change. Because both you and I are water"
Masaru Emoto

CHAPTER FIFTEEN

THE BREATH OF LIFE

"The degree of the vitality of the body and the strength of the barrier to degenerative diseases is in proportion to the ratio of the oxygen saturation of the blood stream, all things being equal."
Kurt Donsbach

There are approximately 75 trillion cells in the human body. (Who do you suppose counted them all?) Each and every one of them requires oxygen for its survival. The average person takes 18,000 to 20,000 breaths every day which consumes approximately 5,000 gallons of air and yet we never think about our breathing. We take our breathing for granted. If we stop breathing, within a few minutes we will die. One does not need a medical degree to understand the vital importance of taking in a breath of fresh air. Therefore, it does not take a rocket scientist to conclude that oxygen must have some significance to life. The quality of the air we breathe and the manner in which we breathe are essential to our well-being, our health, and our life.

Because oxygen is a vital, necessary, prerequisite to life, why hasn't the medical community focused research on oxygen therapy to fend off disease, or better yet, to promote health? We can live without our antacid but we cannot live without oxygen. Oxygen is one of the most powerful weapons we have access to in combating illness. Cancer cells grow in anaerobic conditions. That is, states of low oxygen content. As oxygen levels drop, illness rises and these congesting, stagnating, microbes flourish. When exposed to oxygen therapies these cancer cells do not stand a chance. They will die or even convert back into their original healthy condition as the oxygen rich environment is restored to our tissues.

The response from our aging population to various weather conditions as related to their aches and pains is nature's way of pointing out a remedy. We all know someone who can predict an oncoming storm from their arthritic joints. This is because bad weather is associated with a low pressure system. A low pressure system means oxygen molecules are not as compacted. They are not pressed together tightly. The low atmospheric pressure results in fewer oxygen molecules per cubic inch of space. Therefore, there are fewer oxygen molecules to inhale with each breath. The arthritic cells are suffocating due to a lack of oxygen and the result is pain. Conversely, high pressure systems associated with nice weather deliver a higher concentration of oxygen molecules per cubic inch and consequently are more efficient at feeding the cells with each breath.

Hydrogen concentrates our body's proteins into form. This is called anabolism. (The hydrogenation of peanut butter keeps the oils from separating out. The hydrogenation of margarine gives it its solid form as well.) On the other hand, oxygen reduces the old, used up cells in our body into easily eliminated substances. This is called catabolism. This function of oxygen creates a detoxifying effect in the body. It is a natural cleanser. In this manner, hydrogen puts parts together and creates form while oxygen cleans out the garbage and maintains the mobility of the body. By sweeping up the litter and keeping all the anatomical nooks and crannies free from toxic build up, oxygen keeps us from experiencing the ravages of stiff joints and sluggish organs. When oxygen levels fall, it's purifying role decreases and congestion of the dead cells and toxins increase.

Every cell, and therefore every organ in our body, requires this element for proper function. This is not a debatable statement. We cannot skirt the issue. Deep breathing, whether through physical exercise or focused meditation, infuses the body with life. Oxygen helps eliminate toxins and congestion. It rejuvenates the glands and allows for a more efficient immune system. If someone suffers from chronic infections, deep breathing will help.

By feeding the body this foundation of life, deep breathing will enhance digestion and provide a healthier cardiovascular system. By improving the quality of blood through increasing oxygenation, the heart does not have to work as hard. This can, in turn, extend our life expectancy. One of the best defenses in maintaining vitality is to keep the blood stream clean. The brain requires more oxygen than any other organ. This gift of life fuels the brain and expands consciousness. Proper breathing creates energy, metabolizes food, and enhances all physiological functions. Deep breathing eliminates muscle tension and opens the chest. The catabolic action of oxygen can even help in weight control. Oxygen decreases stress and balances blood pH.

For those of you who still need scientific proof to validate oxygen's potency, we now have it. As recently as April, 2004, science has proven that women with breast cancer have a better survival rate if they exercise. I never doubted the benefits of exercise but I guess science had to once again prove something we all knew. Exactly how does exercise help women with cancer? It is because exercise fills the body with oxygen. Let's take that research one step further and dare make such a bold and sweeping statement. Exercise is beneficial to EVERYONE IN ANY CONDITION, not just women with breast cancer.

Complete obstruction of the airway will cause death within minutes. An acute blockage of oxygen to the brain can cause strokes. Deprive the heart of oxygen and we end up with a heart attack. Without enough oxygen we can fall victim to mental sluggishness, poor memory, depression, and even lose hearing and vision acuity. If oxygen is not completely cut off causing death, but only reduced in its delivery, whether by poor posture, inefficient breathing, smoking, or environmental pollution, our cells will suffer the consequences. All cells, and therefore every organ, are weakened and begin to prematurely degenerate when oxygen demands are not met. Increasing the oxygen levels in our body can only help improve our health regardless of the name of our condition. Any effort to increase the supply of oxygen to our body will pay rich dividends.

"The simplest and most important technique for protecting your health is breathing. I have seen breath control alone achieve remarkable results."
Andrew Weil

We do not think about our breathing yet we do it 24 hours a day. It occurs spontaneously. Because of this, as I mentioned earlier, we tend to take our breathing for granted. But breathing is more than just sucking in air. It is not just something we do to pass the time. Like eating, it is a fundamental process that fosters life. Did you know that there is a right and a wrong way to breathe? We can, indeed, be breathing incorrectly and inefficiently. Are we a chest breather or a belly breather? Do we know the difference? Is breathing merely the physiological act of inhaling and exhaling or is there a deeper spiritual connection? Let's investigate some of these questions in more detail.

Efficient breathing is generated by incorporating the diaphragm. The diaphragm is the muscle of respiration located just under the rib cage. It is a biological gasket that separates the lungs and heart from the organs of digestion. When the diaphragm contracts downward, it creates a vacuum in the chest and air rushes into the lungs and fills the newly created space. The upward motion of the diaphragm then pushes the remaining gas in the lungs back out. Sedentary lifestyles, coupled with poor posture, restrict the diaphragm's ability to fully expand and contract. Without the full incorporation of the diaphragm, we are robbing ourselves of our own health potential. Efficient breathing is incorporated by what is referred to as belly breathing.

When we take a deep breath, our abdomen should actually bulge outward. This is from the downward expansion of the diaphragm. If, instead, we notice our rib cage rising with the in-breath, we are utilizing secondary muscles of respiration. With chest breathing, the muscles of the neck that reach down to the upper rib cage, as well as the muscles of the rib cage and back, are in constant use. This continual strain causes tension within the muscles. Learning to breathe with the diaphragm can ease the chronic tightness we may feel in our back and neck.

Training ourselves to breathe properly can be easy. By lying on our back and placing our hands on top of our abdomen, we can see with each inhalation our resting hands rising and falling with the movement of the diaphragm. Our belly should be doing the physical moving with each breath while our chest, in a sense, just goes along for the ride. Starting our day with a program of ten big, deep belly breaths will get us off to a wonderful start. Energizing the body with oxygen first thing in the morning can clear our head and sharpen our senses. With this, we may even find that our dependency for caffeine can taper off.

There is yet another benefit to belly breathing. The up and down action of the diaphragm massages and squeezes the organs of digestion. This rhythmic pulsing helps to wring out the toxins much like squeezing a sponge. The intermittent pressing action promotes proper blood flow and lymphatic drainage. Deep belly breaths will cause the diaphragm to bear down on and stimulate the intestines. This can aid in relieving constipation and keep the bowel movements regular.

It is indeed a powerfully healing tool when we breathe efficiently and infuse the body with oxygen by utilizing the belly breath. However, there is an even more profound understanding of the act of breathing. Inhaling and exhaling is an overtly conscious, physiological function but it is also an unconscious connection to your spirit. Genesis 2:7 says, "Lord God formed man from the dust of the ground and breathed into his nostrils the breath of life; and man became a living being." This symbolic man (The name Adamah is Hebrew for the ground or dirt) was a lifeless pile of dust until God delivered the animating life force of his breath. Once done, man was born; an entity drawn from the physical earth combined with a spiritual force from heaven. The physical meets the energetic/spiritual. The breath represents our connection to our spirit. If we look up the word spirit in the dictionary, we will see that it comes from the Latin, *spirare*, meaning "to breathe." The breath is the spirit and the spirit is the breath. We breathe in and call it inspiration and we breathe out and call it expiration. In with the spirit and out with the spirit.

"The physical is the substratum of the spiritual, and this fact ought to give to the food we eat, and the air we breathe, a transcendent significance."
William Tyndale

Inspiration and expiration are the means by which we infuse our body not only with physical oxygen but also with the energetic, animating force of the spirit every second of every day. The spirit rides on our breath. The breath, or inspiration, that keeps us alive is the same force that guides us, or inspires us, to our fullest potential. It is no coincidence that an inspiration of breath can cause one to be inspired to greatness. Inspiration of breath creates inspiration for potential.

This focused attention to the breath is exemplified in breathing exercises such as yoga and Tai Chi. Yoga is much more than stretching our tight muscles and trying to assume postures with funny names. Yoga is a Hindu tradition that means to unite. Yoga is the union of our physical self and our spiritual self. As we breathe and move, the spirit, the breath, integrates with all parts of our physical being. The stretching of the physical body allows the spirit to penetrate even deeper into all the nooks and crannies that were once obstructing our awareness to the fullness of life.

Tai Chi refers to the Supreme Force. Tai Chi comes from the Orient and as such, is associated with yin and yang; the notion that duality exists in everything. We have male and female, dawn and dusk, and birth and death. From the standpoint of Tai Chi, yin and yang bring us the dance between the spiritual world and the physical world. The postures and the movements, combined with the focused breath, allows physical man to become more aware of his higher self, his spirit, his potential, or his Supreme Force.

Yoga and Tai Chi seek stillness in movement. These breathing techniques are moving meditations. A Chinese proverb tells us to be as still as a mountain and move like a great river. These statements sound contradictory but they speak of the mindful expression of human form. They are the combination of the intangible spirit and the tangible human. It is the duality that fosters existence. We cannot understand hot unless there is a cold. We cannot appreciate fast unless we experience slow. We cannot feel stillness unless we sense movement. By acknowledging the role of duality, yin and yang, we can comprehend the spirit form only if we have experienced the physical form. Breathing is the tool that bridges the gap between the dualistic qualities of our being. It is the connection that allows our physical body to appreciate and come to know its spiritual side.

When we stop smoking, learn to belly breath, and become active in some focused breathing exercises, we will not only aid the physical body in terms of decreasing muscle tension, lowering blood pressure, curing headaches, and achieve a greater sense of mental clarity, but we will also nourish our spirit as well. We will find it easier to experience joy, peace, and emotional balance. Understanding that breathing is more than just an automatic physiological function and that with every breath we take there is a chance for us to connect with our Supreme Force will help to integrate our body, mind, and spirit to experience its fullest potential.

"Our breathing is the fragile vessel that carries us from life to death."
Frederick Leboyer

CHAPTER SIXTEEN

DO YOU MIND IF I BREATHE WHILE YOU SMOKE?

"Smoking causes lung cancer, heart disease, emphysema, and may complicate pregnancy."
The Surgeon General

Smoking is the second most preventable cause of death and illness in our society (followed by obesity.) Tobacco is responsible for nearly one in five deaths, killing over 400,000 Americans every year. Smoking is responsible for nearly 90% of all lung cancers.[9] Smoking is not just limited to killing humans through the slow, debilitating process of the painful cancer eating away at the flesh. Smoking can kill people in other ways as well. Chronic bronchitis, emphysema, and chronic pulmonary obstructive disease (COPD) are all linked to smoking. The Centers for Disease Control (CDC) states, in their 2002 *Morbidity and Mortality Report,* that nearly 111,000 Americans die from smoking related cardiovascular disease each year. Babies born to smoking mothers are more likely to be born premature and underweight. The white man gave the red man alcohol and the red man, in return, gave the white man tobacco. Sound like a fair trade?

Cigarette smoke contains over 4,000 chemicals including 43 known to cause cancer. Some of these include cyanide, benzene, formaldehyde, methanol (also found in aspartame sweetener), acetylene, ammonia, arsenic, nicotine, toluene, acetone, carbon monoxide, and nitrogen. Smoking is a double edged sword. Every time one inhales a puff of cigarette smoke they not only fill their body with these deadly poisons but also deprive their cells of the life promoting oxygen. They have successfully replaced life with death.

---

[9] CDC.gov/tobacco/factsheets/tobacco_related-mo

If we choose to smoke and are not willing to quit, then we have no one to blame for our health problems but ourselves. When we deprive our body of oxygen, our cells suffer, become weakened, degenerate, and the body develops illness. When we smoke, we introduce poisons such as those found in cigarettes into our body, then we are creating disease. Remember, the four things our body needs to be healthy and live a quality life are nutrition, water, oxygen, and a healthy nervous system.

When we choose to smoke, we choose to deprive our self of the precious life sustaining qualities of oxygen. We choose to suffer the debilitating effects of the cigarette. It is up to each one of us to make this choice on our own. Do we choose health or disease? Life or death?

When I see someone smoking, I see someone who, quite frankly, would rather complain about their health than take responsibility for it. Whether our illness revolves around our skin, bones, pancreas, stomach, sensitivity to pain, immune system, or any other part or function of the body, those cells need oxygen to live and smoking will not supply them with one microscopic bit of it. Because of its toxic makeup, cigarettes will only make health concerns worse by robbing the body of what it needs the most. I will not accept the excuse of addiction. If we smoke and have health care concerns, we need to make a choice. Do we continue to deprive ourselves of oxygen and live with the ever debilitating effects of chronic disease or do we find the strength to quit and begin to appreciate the subtle joys found in improving the quality of our life? Everything we do is a choice we must take responsibility for.

"Smokers, male and female, inject idleness and excuse in their lives every time they light a cigarette."
Sidonie Colette

CHAPTER SEVENTEEN

COUCH POTATOES AND IDIOT BOXES

"Those who think they have no time for bodily exercise will sooner or later have to find time for illness."
Edward Stanley

There are many levels of fitness. There is the weekend athlete, the routine workout, the professional athlete, and Olympic conditioning. There are just as many supposed reasons to exercise. "I want to get rid of my middle aged spread," the "I want to look good at the beach," and then there is the New Year's resolution of, "This is the year I want to lose twenty pounds." Whatever our level of exercise and whatever our reason to exercise, there is but one underlying physiological effect. That is to infuse our body and all its cells with oxygen. I don't care what name they apply to our workout routine, or which exercise fad is currently sweeping the country, or what celebrity endorsed fitness machine is coming through our television, the bottom line is simply that exercise fills our body with oxygen.

When we put our body under physical exertion for a prolonged period of time, the oxygen demands from within increase and make us breathe harder and deeper. Breathing harder and deeper expands the chest, invigorates the organs, and saturates the tissues with oxygen. Sitting on the couch, lying in bed, or endlessly surfing the internet will do nothing to saturate our body with the life giving essence of oxygen. Granted, exercise can help us lose weight, add muscle tone and muscle mass, increase metabolism, and clear the mind, but none of that will happen without oxygen.

Exercising does not mean we have to spend exorbitant monthly fees at some flashy, neon riddled health club that locks us into a two year contract knowing we will not last more than six months there. We do not have to succumb to the flashy television ads that boast six pack abs, tight derrieres wrapped in spandex, and large breasts. (I am not quite sure how silicone implants relate to fitness centers.) We do not need to bench press 200 pounds to be healthy. We do not need to be able to run a mile in under five minutes and we do not need to spend 60 minutes trying to keep up with the advanced dance class masquerading as a beginner's aerobics session. These are certainly admirable traits and congratulations to those who can. However, they are not necessary to achieve lasting health benefits from exercise.

This is not to say that exercising to that level of intensity is bad. I applaud those who put in an effort to reshape their bodies. They have set fitness goals and are proactive in their health choices. Aerobic conditioning is a positive venture. It can create a strong, efficient heart and an increased lung capacity. Strong muscles, including the heart, will go a long way in preserving the youthful condition of the body. All of the body's processes will respond more efficiently and effectively with routine exercise as a stimulant. The level of exercise will obviously need to match the fitness goals we have set. Again, we do not need to dedicate hours each day to a fitness regimen to obtain beneficial results. It takes very little effort to rework our schedule and add some easy exercises to our daily routine.

Life is motion and motion is life. The key here is to add some movement to our life. We need to get out from in front of the television or computer and move our body. For those of us who wish to live in a politically correct environment, I will tell you that Americans have become too sedentary and too comfortable with modernized technology. For those of us who appreciate a more straight forward approach I can inform you that there are too many lazy people in America. Fifty million adults are obese. That, my friends, is just not acceptable. Being overweight is estimated to cause

325,000 deaths each year.[10] Obesity is also one of the reasons why health insurance costs are out of reach for so many Americans. Obesity contributes its own form of magnification to our health issues. Obesity has been directly related to heart disease, diabetes, high cholesterol, and high blood pressure. As the numbers of obese Americans grows, so too does the number of doctor visits and insurance claims. With insurance companies inundated with mountains of claims, they are forced to increase their rates to keep up with the reimbursement demands. What if we focused on the obese Americans with high blood pressure, high cholesterol, heart disease, and diabetes, and convinced them to add a mile of walking to the end of their day? Could we begin to create healthier Americans which could have the potential to decrease doctor's office visits and therefore reduce the insurance claim load dramatically? An exercise program, of even the smallest degree, is missing from too many households and the health and well-being of this country is feeling the burden. In 2000, the estimated annual cost of obesity in the United States was around $117 billion.[11]

Too many Americans circle the supermarket in their cars waiting for a parking space to open up near the front door. Too many Americans choose to ride the escalator at the mall and the elevator at work instead of walking up one flight of stairs. We can now run a great majority of our errands and never leave the car. We drive up to the bank teller, drive up to the mailbox at the post office, and then drive through some fast food joint for lunch. There are drive-through pharmacies and we can get the oil changed in our car without ever leaving the comfort of the driver's seat. We even have the Segway, a two wheeled scooter contraption that moves

---

[10] David Allison et al, "Annual Deaths Attributed to Obesity in the United States," *Journal of American Medical Association*. 1999;282: p. 1530-1538.

[11] U.S. Department of Agriculture. www.csrees.usda.gov

us from place to place without taking a step. We have children old enough to walk but are instead being pushed in strollers through the mall. If we insist on not using our legs and lungs, evolution may be forced to change us back into fish.

The advent of the internet has given us the capacity to search out the remotest corners of the world for information, acquire cheap tickets to airlines and motels, sell and buy things, email our friends and family, bank on line and so much more. It has also created a generation of internet addicts who spend hours of mindless button pushing instead of mowing the lawn or walking the dog. We have children who will spend hours gazing at the latest DVD playing on the television instead of going outside and riding their bicycles. We have created a generation of zombies who would rather play video games than shovel the snow from the front walkway.

"Lack of activity destroys the good condition of every human being, while movement and methodical exercise save it and preserve it."
Plato

The challenge for us here is to increase the exercise level of our every day routine. We can start by purchasing a pedometer. They are inexpensive and a handy tool to gauge our level of movement. Each day go about your business as normal as possible. Use the pedometer and record the number of steps taken at the end of each day. Take off the pedometer while you are at home. Walking in the house from room to room does not count. Calculate the average number of steps for each day. If our number is not 10,000 or more, we have room to improve. For most of us there is lots of room for improvement.

Please do not fret and become depressed. We can easily reach 10,000 steps each day with very little added effort. Here is how. Never ever use a drive up for anything. Get out of the car and walk to the bank teller inside. Walk into the post office to drop off the mail. If we must eat out we need to walk into the restaurant to get our food. And we can't just park our car near the front door either. That would defeat the purpose of the exercise routine. We must park our car a good distance from the front door. Whether grocery shopping or heading into work, we must choose the parking space furthest from the building. We are not in so much of a rush that an extra five minutes of walking each day will set our life back. We have the time and we need the movement. Never take the escalator or elevator to go up a few flights. Head for the stairs. Be diligent at adding extra steps to the day for one week and then compare your pedometer numbers. We can easily add 1,500 to 2,000 more steps each day without a change in routine, just a change in approach.

If we are still under the goal of 10,000 steps per day, the challenge continues. For every American who does not now have a regular exercise program of some sort established in their daily routine, now is the time to start. Again, this can be done with very little change to our routine. We do not need to commit several hours each day to venture off to the nearest fitness center.

First, we are to cut our television viewing time down to ten hours per week. I bet you think that ten hours is a lot of television watching and that there is no way someone would even come close to that much viewing. To the contrary, I'll bet that most Americans (remember, there are 50 million obese adults in the country) are glued to the television set from 6:00 at night until you go to bed around 11:00. That's five hours each day and probably more on the weekends. This equates to 25-40 hours of television each week. Ten hours of television each week allows us twenty, half hour programs. That's more than enough. Pick your favorite shows and limit your television time to just those. I will even sweeten the deal and allow one extra movie rental each week on top of the ten hours of television.

The extra time not spent in front of the television can be used to walk around the block. Pick up a game of tennis with a friend, shoot some hoops at the park, ride our bicycle, mow the lawn, go ice skating, or toss the football in the back yard with our children. None of this requires a membership to a health club and all of it benefits the body. Get out in the sun and fresh air and move. By adding such simple exercise routines to our day, our muscles will become stronger, our joints will move with more ease, and our metabolism will increase. Our heart and lungs will thank us as oxygen is carried through the vascular system with greater ease and efficiency. Every cell in our body will be able to breathe a sigh of relief (literally and figuratively) as the new infusion of oxygen cleans, invigorates, and nourishes them.

By adding steps to our normal daily chores and replacing television watching with some form of movement, we can achieve a level of 10,000 steps each day without much effort. For those Americans who have become extremely sedentary, you may need to start slow and set goals. We have nothing to lose except aches and pains, multiple trips to the doctor's office, and inches on our waistline. We have everything to gain including a new appreciation for life, stronger muscles, a greater ease of motion, and a healthy outlook on life.

"Walking is man's best medicine."
Hippocrates

CHAPTER EIGHTEEN

CHIROPRACTIC: THE BEST KEPT SECRET ON EARTH

"Disease of every organ or portion of the body may, and very frequently do, arise from defects in the nerve centers rather than the organ itself."
Daniel David Palmer

The fourth factor in obtaining health, but no less important than nutrition, water, and oxygen is the need for an animating source of energy. We all have an animating source of energy or we would not be alive. This is that magic *something* that combines our food, water, and oxygen into a living, breathing, thinking, moving form. There is that *something* that has sparked our elements into life. We can hook up an oxygen tank to a cadaver, put an apple in its stomach, and pour water into its mouth but that will not bring the cadaver to life. There is still one missing element.

Our car can have a full tank of premium gasoline, a fresh oil change, and a clean carburetor but unless there is a spark to ignite the mixture nothing will happen. This special *something*, this animating life force in our body, has been described through time by every culture, in every language, on every continent.

Each primitive clan or tribe would use their own personal beliefs, seasonal constraints, and spiritual concepts to mold a distinct idea as to where this life force originates from, how it transforms into matter, and how to address it. Though the mythologies created to explain this phenomenon are different, they all relate to the same thing. There is some mysterious *something* somewhere that has created life as we know it. Some refer to this energetic force as chi, kundalini, or prana. Other cultures acknowledge a divine creator or God as the animating force of life. This Creator has been called many things through eons of time and multitudes of cultures. We may or may not be familiar with names such as Brahma, Wankan Tonka, Yahweh, Jehovah, Allah, Gitchi Manito, or Vishnu. We can define it how we would like, as to make ourselves comfortable with our paradigm but we cannot discredit the underlying basic concept. There is a magical force, a *something*, that moves life. The secret to health lies in how well this life giving energy flows through our body without interference.

So what does all this talk of God and the many names attributed to this power have to do with chiropractic medicine? Keep reading and I promise to make the connection soon.

When people speak of chiropractors they often refer to them as back doctors. The majority of Americans have come to understand and accept that chiropractors can help relieve back pain. They may even dare venture to the chiropractor's office in an attempt to find relief from chronic headaches, sciatica, whiplash, or some other musculoskeletal ailment. While chiropractic can certainly help these conditions, limiting the potential of the chiropractic adjustment in this manner is analogous to using only one syllable words to communicate. In doing so, we will be missing out on the infinite potential of each.

These limitations of chiropractic have been created and established not by those who understand chiropractic's basic philosophy but by those who fear the truth inherent in the principles of its discovery. Chiropractic medicine is much more than any definition can encompass. It is more than a physical asymmetry, a muscle spasm, or a misaligned spine. It is a healing modality that cannot be pigeon holed into categories or techniques. Chiropractic medicine is a healing art in contact with the Big Picture. But as long as the medical and pharmaceutical establishments control the governing bodies that dictate health care, the truth about chiropractic will remain one of the best kept secrets on earth.

Before we explore the spiritual side of chiropractic health care, I want to give you a brief history lesson. (Hey, it's better than a physics lesson, isn't it?) Doctor Daniel David Palmer, the founder of chiropractic, was born on March 7, 1845, in Toronto, Canada. He had been a self-taught magnetic healer nearly a decade prior to his discovering the principles that comprise the chiropractic healing art. Magnetic healing and other forms of vibrational medicine are just now, over 150 years later, beginning to come of age. Dr. Palmer was well ahead of his time.

However, there are still those in the medical profession whose focus it is to live in a closed box and debase chiropractic. They love to characterize Dr. Palmer as a quack and therefore discredit the whole profession. They are quick to point out the non-scientific sham of magnetic healing forgetting that in the late 1800's all of scientific medicine was in its infancy. There was the snake oil salesman venturing from town to town with his wagon load of potions, and Mary Baker Eddy had just begun her initiation of Christian Science. Doctor Mesmer's form of hypnosis therapy was new to this country and Andrew Still was developing osteopathy. It was a time filled with questions and those pioneers brave enough to try and find the answers.

Not only is Dr. Palmer's education constantly questioned, for he was by and large self-taught, but his prior vocation as a fish salesman is forever being dredged through the anti-chiropractic propaganda. To add insult to injury, Dr. Palmer is not even given the dignity of being called a salesman or grocer. He is referred to as a fish monger. The manipulation of this small adjective creates a whole new characterization of him. What could an uneducated fish monger ever know about the human condition? This all to discredit Dr. Palmer's ability of ever being able to express an idea that differs from the reigning paradigm and contribute anything of value to the community, let alone the world. I suppose we are to believe once a fish salesman, always a fish salesman. If that were the case, a lanky man from Kentucky who worked on the railroads could never become the President of the United States an abolish slavery. Fortunately for us, the greatness of a man cannot be limited by those who judge him. Dr. Palmer knew that this level of greatness can only be limited by he who seeks it.

In 1895, in Davenport, Iowa, chiropractic was born. While examining Harvey Lillard, a deaf janitor in the building in which Dr. Palmer worked, Dr. Palmer noticed that Harvey had a vertebra in his back that did not line up with the others. As legend has it, Dr. Palmer "wracked" the vertebra back into position. When Harvey rose from the table, he could hear the clacking of horse's hooves on the cobblestone street below the open window. His hearing had been restored. Shortly after Harvey's relief from deafness, Dr. Palmer had a similar case involving a heart condition. Two diseases, so dissimilar, that were improved after spinal manipulation must have a common ground. This common ground was found to be nerve tension and the cure was created through the chiropractic adjustment.

"Look well to the spine for it is the requisite for many diseases."
Hippocrates

This is how simple the chiropractic tenets are: The nervous system is comprised of our brain, spinal cord and all the nerves that branch from the cord and traverse the openings between our vertebrae. These nerves branch like roots of a tree and weave their way through the entire body. Our brain is the master computer of our being and it runs the business of our life by sending and receiving messages through the spinal cord, out the nerves and to all the organs, tissues, joints, and assorted parts of our body. The nervous system allows every cell in our body the direction or guidance it needs to adapt to its surroundings by not only communicating directly with the cells but also by supplying them a bioelectrical spark to ignite the cells into action. The nervous system is our anatomical phone company as well as the biological electric company. It is the role of this nervous system to control, coordinate, and regulate *every* (Yes, I did say *every*) function of the human body. Without our nervous system intact and operating we are no different than a corpse.

    The squeezing of the intestines to move along the digested matter is controlled by the nervous system. The collapsing of the diaphragm which allows air to rush into our lungs is controlled by the nervous system. The release of bile from the gall bladder, insulin from the pancreas, and adrenalin from the adrenal glands is all under direct supervision of the nervous system. Hormones regulate function as well but our hormones ultimately originate from specific organs that are directly stimulated by the nervous system. Without our nervous system our stomach does not digest, our liver does not balance cholesterol, and our muscles do not contract to allow us to put our arms around our children.

    Our mouth cannot produce saliva, nor can we create neurotransmitters, antihistamines, cortisone, or new bone cells to mend a fracture unless our nervous system is operating properly. I need to repeat here that EVERY function of your body is controlled, coordinated, and regulated by the nervous system! If our insulin does not control our sugar levels, look to the nervous system. If our respiratory system does not coordinate itself with the seasons, look to the nervous system. If our blood pressure does not regulate correctly, look to the nervous system.

Action potential is the phrase used to describe the electrical impulse of communicating energy that travels through the nerves. This wave of biological information is much like a pluck of a guitar string. When the guitar string is too tight or too loose, the note we hear when the string is hit sounds out of key. The frequency of the cord is off. The action potential, though infinitely more complex, can align itself with the guitar string analogy. If the nerve is too tense or too slack, the frequency of the action potential is changed. The electrical message traveling through the nerve as action potential is altered. Without proper nerve tension allowing proper action potential, organ function becomes aberrant. The target organ is not receiving its proper bioelectrical impulse and therefore does not operate properly. Too much tension in a nerve/action potential will create excitation (stomach ulcer for example) and too much slack in the nerve/action potential will create sluggishness (indigestion). The state of disease depends upon which nerves are too slack and which nerves are too tense. It is nerve tension that is the basis of functional activity and the difference between health and disease. By manipulating the bones of the back, or any bone of the body for that matter, a skilled chiropractor can influence the tension on the nerves and restore the action potential to its proper frequency.

"It is not for chiropractors to try to improve the basic law- this is impossible- but to remove any obstructions brought about by perversions of that law, to the further end of a greater and freer expression is what the law of cycles demands in every phase and attribute."
R. W. Stephenson

Weather we are a librarian, rock musician, author, or a soccer mom, the nervous system has the same functions for everyone. When chiropractic is insulted and our philosophy attacked, I have to wonder what kind of education the medical students are getting at Harvard. This is basic physiology. I cannot understand how one can graduate from a medical school and not appreciate the interconnectedness of the nervous system to the health of the body. Even the AMA's Home Medical Encyclopedia, written for the common folk, states that the nervous system is the body's information-gathering, storage, and control system. The encyclopedia continues to say, "The overall function of the nervous system is to gather information about the external environment and the body's internal state, to analyze this information, and to initiate appropriate responses." With that definition, why hasn't medicine put more focus on the state of the nervous system as a factor in health?

If our bowels are not eliminating waste matter appropriately, our nervous system could be at fault. If the ovaries are not producing estrogen and progesterone in the proper ratios, the nervous system may be at fault. It would make sense then to look to the controlling mechanism within the body. That master controlling mechanism can only be our nervous system.

Now I must ask, can headaches be related to the ability of our nervous system to regulate some bodily function? Why do some people suffer from headaches and I do not? Is it because some people are somehow deficient in aspirin? Did they not get their RDA of Tylenol? Wait! There is no RDA for Tylenol. Why does my body adapt to changes without producing a headache and theirs does not? Maybe there is something inherently wrong with their system of adaptation. Can it be that their nervous system is under stress and therefore the action potential is altered so that it cannot create the proper changes in their body that they need to adapt to the new condition? Could it really be that simple? Yes it can.

Who tolerates severe menstrual cramps because they only incapacitate them for a few days each month?

Who blames their thyroid for slow metabolism? Who has to pop a few pills before they eat a spicy meal? How many people suffer from asthma, ADD, high blood pressure, chronic fatigue, ear infections, or fibromyalgia? These are all signs of the body not being able to comprehend its environment internally as well as externally and that is a direct function of the nervous system. The body is not able to express its inherent state of perfection. Perfection you ask? Are we really supposed to believe that our bodies are perfectly designed?

Consider the miracle that we are for just a moment. At conception, we are but one single cell. That cell divided into two cells and those two cells divided into four. This process continues until such a time when the cells are ready to differentiate. That is, they start to become specialized. Some cells will develop into our eyes and create vision. Some cells will become the connective tissue of the Achilles tendon while still other will turn into the white blood cells that participate in the immune system. Some cells become hair while others form into our eardrums; All unique to a specific function, all in their right places, and all without the necessity of medical intervention. This formation of life doesn't need FDA approval or medical legislation. It is perfect all by itself.

"There is simply the rose; it is perfect in every moment of its existence."
Ralph Waldo Emerson

When these cells start to specialize, which system is the first to evolve? Is it the heart? Lungs? Maybe it is the eyes? It is none of these. The first system to differentiate and develop is the nervous system; the spinal cord and the brain. I will even go so far as to theorize that before these cells differentiate, when they are still just a conglomerate of identical cells, that they are even then nervous tissue. Science just hasn't been able to detect it as such. This cellular differentiation into neural tissue is merely the first recognizable form of the nervous system. Why does this tissue form before all others? The answer is easy. Remember, it is the function of the nervous system to control, coordinate and regulate *every* function of the human body. This includes directing the development of our very being right from conception. This is why I believe undifferentiated cells must be coded with nervous tissue instruction. Our conception is our nervous system.

When something goes wrong in a company who is ultimately responsible? It is of course the CEO. The CEO must be aware of every operation under his/her control. In the case of our body manifesting health or disease, that CEO is our nervous system. With this in mind, chiropractic becomes not just medicine for back pain, numbness, migraines, or carpal tunnel. Chiropractic is not merely relegated to pain relief, HMO participation, or a label of alternative health care. Chiropractic is not about a short leg, bulging disc, or pinched nerve. It is more than a physical asymmetry, a muscle spasm, or a misaligned spine. It is our ability to comprehend life and design physiologically appropriate responses to changes imposed upon it.

Without a reminder scribbled on a post-it note, the nervous system adjusts our blood pressure to accommodate sitting, standing, or lying down. It instinctively raises our hand to swat away an errant projectile. Without complaint, the body replaces dead skin cells with new ones. Within the community of cells that come together to create life there are no criminals, no hateful thugs, and no gangsters. There is only the will to translate the Breath of Life into flesh and blood.

I cannot accept the theories of diseases caused by genes for genes are inherently endowed with the principles that create and propagate life. If we invented an automobile that ran on water, would we also create a self-destruct mechanism inside the engine? How can we come to believe that an omnipotent, omniscient, creative force that produced life as we know it would program this work of art with defective pieces? Plain and simple, God doesn't make junk. The very definition of life itself rules out the genetic defect theory. Every living creature on earth has the desire to propagate its own species and that is life promoting, not life demoting. Medicine is quick to blame our genes for every ailment in which they cannot find a cause for. They cannot find a cause for so many diseases because they are looking in the wrong places for answers. Medical science stares at genes and declares that disease must be in there somewhere. If they looked closer at the nervous system and its role in the Big Picture, they would indeed find a true cause of disease.

That spark of life, originating in the hands of God, flowing from above to down and from inside to outside is consigned to the structures we call the nervous system. This very framework enables us to hear the purr of a kitten, view a rose bedecked with dew, and feel the wet sand from the shoreline slip between our toes. The nervous system is the greatest magician on earth as it can recast a green pepper into human life by merely tickling the digestive system with action potential. The anatomy we call the nervous system is responsible for accepting the Creator's inspiration for perfection and transforming it into physical existence. We hold this anatomy accountable for directing the orchestra of our lives. It tells the heart to beat, the kidneys to filter, and the blood vessels to constrict and dilate. It tastes the sour berries and feels the warmth of the sun on our faces. It sparks our legs to ambulation. It smells the cinnamon. This precious entity that we call the nervous system is the interface that moves human experience. Chiropractic is a healing art that dances with that part of our anatomy in which the very force of life is transformed into matter. It is our breath, our thoughts, our passion, our life. It is the modality that speaks both languages of spirit and body. Our nervous system is the metaphor that binds spirit and heaven into matter and earth. Our nervous system now becomes much more than just some piece of our anatomy that can be dissected for the sake of a text book. We chiropractors, by adjusting the bones of the spine and extremities, set free the incarcerated impulse of consciousness that sweeps through the nerves and animates every cell of our being.

The reality of life is a luxurious quilting of interwoven layers reaching through and connecting the spirit to the soul to the mind and to the body. Though each layer may have its own characteristics, they are all one in the same. Albert Einstein proposed that matter and energy are just different forms of the same expression. This implies that the biological realms are the spiritual realms and visa-versa. The human experience is spirit in physical form. Spirit may descend into matter but the matter is spirit nonetheless. The nervous system, in all its mystical, magical glory, therefore becomes the first physical evidence we have of God's inspiration for human perfection. Our nervous system is the hard drive that translates our divine program into a human program.

When people seek out a chiropractor for an alignment they are not merely aligning their physical structures to relieve stress from their muscles, bones, and nerves. Though that is definitely a good idea, it is not the Big Picture. The Big Picture includes spirit. We will receive an alignment alright but it is an alignment with our life's purpose. By releasing the nervous system from stress we are reconnecting with the perfection that is our self and always will be. As all of nature is bound by certain cycles, patterns and laws, so too is our existence and that existence is controlled, coordinated, and regulated by our nervous system. The chiropractic adjustment is about removing the barriers that inhibit our physical expression with its true source. The adjustment will liberate the nervous system, and therefore our spirit, from the stranglehold of dis-ease (not being at ease with one's self) and allow our body's innate intelligence to once again manifest through our flesh and blood. Chiropractic, like other true forms of healing, is a manipulation of the spirit as it manifests through matter.

> *"There is but one cause in disease, the body's inability to comprehend itself and its environment. There is but one cure in disease, the body's ability to heal itself. And there is only one thing any doctor can do for a patient and that is to remove an obstruction to healing thus facilitating it."*
> Fred H. Barge

Textbooks told us chiropractic students that the misaligned vertebra was called a subluxation. That is a misalignment of a joint less than a dislocation. Look deeper into the word subluxation. Lux is Latin for light. Sub means below or less than. A subluxation is a manifestation of a condition that is less than pure light. As we remove subluxations we are literally letting the light shine through. Is that something this country is ready for, or do we feel more secure just accepting chiropractic as back pain relief?

There is nothing enlightening about misalignments, imbalances, or subluxations. The living organism does not function according to medical school departments, vaccine schedules, or pharmaceutical intervention. It functions according to God's will and it is directed through the brilliant dictation of the nervous system. It is said that our life is God's gift to us and what we do with it is our gift back to God. Don't let a subluxation interfere with that.

The chiropractic adjustment is a telescopic connection to the Big Picture. Removing subluxations restores life not by replacing with implants, controlling with machines, or chemically altering with drugs, but rather by allowing, freeing, and innately accepting the ability of the body to regulate itself. The chiropractic philosophy is hopeful of possibilities and pursues what is right within the body, not fearful of probabilities searching for what is wrong within the body. Exalting the Hippocratic tradition of "first do no harm," chiropractic exercises the body's wisdom in contrast to exorcizing the body's failures. Chiropractic moves by experience, intuition, and spirit, not by scientific dogma and outdated tradition, for the miracle of life cannot be truly explained scientifically. One cannot dissect love, grow the breath in a laboratory, or capture the sunshine in a test tube. Chiropractic focuses on health not disease, the whole body not parts, and promotes life rather than avoids death.

The proof that chiropractic is a legitimate healing art can be found in the fact that it exists and continues to do so in spite of the overwhelming opposition by the medical community. Chiropractic has stood in the flames of slander and libel for over 115 years and has lived to tell its own story. What established chiropractic as the largest natural healing art in this country was not its relatively small lobby groups or its national associations but rather its ability to create clinical success stories out of medical failures. By adhering to the tenets of nature's perfection, the patient heals what was once declared incurable. Chiropractic is not part of medicine and was never meant to be. It is a philosophical approach to life that is bound by the laws of nature.

"The doctor of the future will give no medicine, but will interest his patients in the care of the human frame, in diet, and in the cause and prevention of disease."
Thomas Edison

CHAPTER NINETEEN

VACCINES: A TOXIC SHOT SYNDROME

"At two in the morning, she had been crying for thirteen hours and her fever was 105 degrees. By the third morning she was still screaming. I couldn't believe that this was a normal reaction to the DPT no matter what my pediatrician kept telling me."
From the book, A Shot in the Dark

Medical errors have certainly been etched into our history books. George Washington was bled to death by his physicians. Mercury at one time was used as a curative. Tonsils were irradiated. Hysterectomies were performed to keep women from acting out of line or seemingly being "hysterical." Many practices have been found to be erroneous when, at one time, they were accepted procedure. Doctor Semmelweis was chastised by his peers when he suggested that his colleagues wash their hands between the acts of delivering babies and performing surgeries. Vaccination will one day be just another example of misguided medicine. Ouch! That's a pretty bold statement. I am not alone in that thought, however. Here is why I believe this way.

As students at Palmer College of Chiropractic, we were continuously influenced by the inspirational thoughts and philosophical writings of Dr. B. J. Palmer, the son of the founder of chiropractic. Generations before me were blessed with his wisdom through chiropractic epithets painted on the walls throughout the entire school. Unfortunately, pressure from the medical model to and conform to their paradigm standards forced Palmer College to "clean up" its act. Most of the wall writings were painted over. Still, you can hear the spirit of Dr. Palmer walking the halls chanting, "The power that made the body heals the body. It happens no other way." With this kind of indoctrination, I was left standing in a quandary. My life growing up was filled with the propaganda that insisted if we did not meet our proper vaccination schedules we would have a greater risk of catching one or more of the so called deadly childhood diseases. The same was true with antibiotics. Both were as much a part of life as summer picnics and school dances. While attending Palmer College, I was suddenly confronted with this conflicting information. Medicine demanded that we cling to vaccines and antibiotics with the same passion that we used to cling to our neonatal placenta. However, the chiropractic philosophy is the complete antithesis to the idea of artificially induced immunity. So what was I to believe?

I confronted one of my teachers with this dilemma. Her answer was not an answer at all but a challenge to introduce myself to the school's library system and investigate the vaccine issue for myself. Dr. Maxine McMullen had just started me out on what was to become not only the very beginnings of this book but also one of the most important lessons of my life.

Dr. Palmer's legacy was telling me that there were options regarding childhood diseases and alternatives regarding life and death. During my researching stint in the library, what caught my attention more than anything else was that even if one did not wish to embody the chiropractic philosophy and lifestyle, vaccination stood all by itself as a bad idea. The information I found while doing my research was not necessarily pro-chiropractic. What I discovered was the idea that the need for vaccinations to spare us from childhood diseases was a farce. It is a lie propagated upon the people without the opportunity for resistance. It is a no questions asked faith based money making enterprise. These are strong words, I know, but after you are exposed to the information that I found, you too may find truth in my castigations.

One of the most compelling facts about the

efficacy of vaccinations deals with the rate of demise of the childhood diseases before their respective vaccines were ever disseminated. Medicine has us convinced that vaccines are the sole reason for the eradication of measles, mumps, pertussis, and the like. However, when we compare morbidity and mortality rates (sickness and death) of infectious disease, we will find that these diseases were all well on their way to disappearing on their own even before the vaccine was ever in mass usage.

In 1901, the total number of deaths due to measles was 11,956. In 1956, the measles death total was reduced to 203. By 1955, before the first measles shot was ever given, the death rate had declined nearly 98% on its own. Diphtheria had a similar decrease in death rate from 48,839 in 1901 to 1135 in 1941 before any vaccine for it appeared.[12] The four leading causes of death from 1911 to 1945 in children ages 1-14 years old were diphtheria, measles, scarlet fever, and whooping cough. That may not come as a surprise, but a closer look at the statistics will. According to the Metropolitan Life Insurance Company's *Health Progress*, in 1948, the combined death rate from these diseases declined 95% on their own before mass immunization began in the United States.

Whooping cough (pertussis), all on its own, followed the same decline in incidence prior to the introduction of its vaccine. Most of this information has never been spelled out in this manner. One has to be able to read between the lines of the research and documentation. For example, the 1989 *American Medical Association Home Medical Encyclopedia*, states, "Before the introduction of a vaccine against pertussis in the 1950's, this disease killed more children every year in the US than all other infectious diseases

---

[12] Michael Alderson, International Mortality Statistics. New York, NY: Facts on File, Inc., 1981. pp 163-189, 313.

combined." It is followed by this graph.

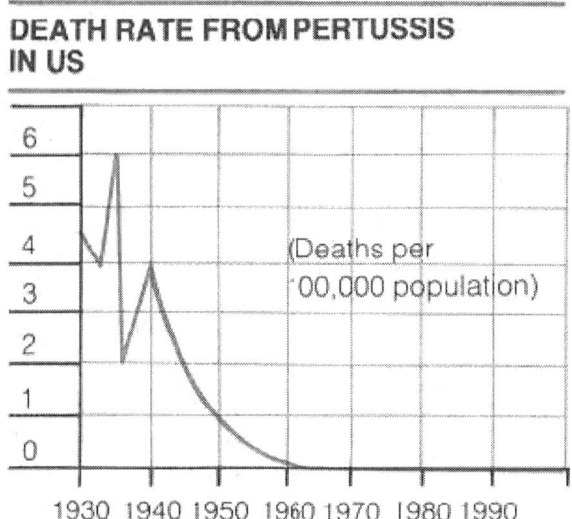

The decline of pertussis
Pertussis caused thousands of deaths annually in the 1930s and 1940s. Now there are just a handful of deaths each year.

Do you see the contradiction? According to the AMA's own chart, the death rate from 1935 to 1950 dropped from 6/100,000 to 1/100,000 all on its own prior to the advent of the vaccine. This AMA admission, though they did not intend it to be such, is in itself powerful medicine in the acknowledgment of the truth concerning vaccine's role in eliminating infectious disease. This kind of data is readily available to anyone who wishes to dig for it.

The total death rate from pertussis declined from 33,094 in 1901 to 1460 in 1946 without one vaccine ever being given.[13]

Faced with this kind of information, medicine still credits the vaccine machine for defeating death. No artificial replacement for our naturally acquired immunity could ever equate to these kinds of decreases in infectious disease rates.

Polio is still fresh in the minds of my parent's generation and, as expected, when I give a lecture on vaccinations I am confronted by those wonderful, silver haired Doubting Thomases. They seem to be able to accept my inquisition on vaccines up until I begin to critique the polio epidemic. I contend that much of the statistical information concerning polio was exaggerated due to the President himself, Franklin Roosevelt, being confined to a wheelchair from the disease.

In 1952, the government began a subsidized study of polio. Not surprisingly, every diagnosed case of polio became a money maker for the hospitals and the incidence of polio skyrocketed. Doctor Mendelsohn stated in his book, *Confessions of a Medical Heretic*, that during the time of this subsidized study, "everything from stiff necks to sprained ankles became a case of polio." In 1921 there were 7229 deaths in the U.S. due to polio. This number fell to 1604 deaths by 1956.[14] The polio vaccine was not used on a grand scale until then. If the polio vaccine was allegedly responsible for the decline of polio infection in the U.S., why did the epidemics of Europe also end where the polio vaccine was not so widely in use?

I have pointed out many times in this book that when man violates Natural Law he creates his own problems. Perhaps the polio epidemic of the late 1940s to the mid-1950s was marked by a decrease in breast

---

[13] Michael Alderson.
[14] Michael Alderson.

feeding as mothers opted for the baby bottle. Mother's milk contains a neutralizing agent that inactivates the polio virus. Does this help explain a rise in polio rates during the same period? Given the fact that before the vaccine was introduced the polio virus could be found virtually everywhere, natural immunity was already as close to being as global as it could ever be. Who should take credit for the decline in polio related deaths, natural resistance or vaccines?

To help propagate the success of the polio vaccine, diseases were redefined and the statistics were manipulated. After the introduction of the Salk vaccine, the definition of an epidemic changed from 20 cases per 100,000 population to 35 cases per 100,000 population. That game of semantics alone would cause a decrease in the rate of epidemics. Prior to 1954, for a diagnosis of paralytic polio, the patient had to exhibit the symptoms for only 24 hours. With the advent of the vaccine, in order to be classified as paralytic polio the patient had to exhibit the paralytic symptoms for at least 60 days.[15] When medicine changes the definition of an epidemic and changes the definition of the disease, they can change the course of history without ever administering one vaccine shot.

If vaccines saved us from the ruthless onslaught of infectious disease, what ever happened to scarlet fever, typhus, and, until recently, chicken pox, for which there were no vaccines? Where are those epidemics? Their rates of infection have all decreased on their own without the advent of a vaccine.

That kind of information alone was enough to convince me that the creation of vaccines was an inept attempt for medicine to create a savior for a world that didn't need one. I also knew that I had just scratched the tip of the iceberg as far as the suppression of the truth was concerned. If vaccines are such an inspiration to

---

[15] Hearings on H.R. 10541, pp. 94, 96.

health, why are they the only medicine forced upon us by law? Shouldn't they stand on their own merits? If the government was giving away free gold, diamonds, or BMWs, the people of this country would be standing in line to get their fair share. We understand the value of them. The fact that George Washington was a great leader and helped a bunch of ill-equipped farmers defeat the world's strongest army does not need to be propagandized. His legend has stood the test of time. So why can't vaccines stand on their own merit without the pressure from organized medicine and why are they mandated by legal scripture?

Maybe you concede, from the information given above, that naturally acquired immunity to infectious childhood diseases was well on its way to becoming complete before their respective vaccines were introduced. Maybe you are thinking that vaccines at least helped out at the tail end of the disease cycle. Maybe you think vaccines supported our immune system so that our defenses did not have to work so hard. Sorry, think again. Vaccines actually cause more stress within our body's defense system. The truth is that vaccines are made from synthetic chemicals and poisons and therefore cannot contribute to our health in any way. I know, you don't believe me, right? How can the medical profession promote and distribute poisons under the guise of health? All we have to do is read the ingredient label on any package insert or look up the information in the PDR (Physicians Desk Reference) and we will see the truth.

If we did, we would see such toxins as formaldehyde usually disguised as formalin. It's mainly used to disinfect the vaccine. However, its inability to disinfect immediately became apparent. Only two months into the Salk campaign, the U.S. Public Health Service, on June 23, 1955, announced that there had been 168 confirmed cases of poliomyelitis among the vaccinated with six deaths. An Associated Press

Dispatch from Boston on August 30, 1955, reported 2,027 cases of polio in Massachusetts, against 273 at the same time the previous year representing an increase of 743%.[16] State after state began reporting increases in polio and paralytic polio cases. Not long after the first Salk polio vaccine was injected into American children, paralysis increased about 50% from 1957 to 1958, and about 80% from 1958 to 1959. Formaldehyde is designated by the EPA as a hazardous substance and it is a known carcinogen yet the FDA allows the drug companies to use it in our children's vaccines. How does formaldehyde promote health?

Other toxins used in the preparation of the exalted vaccine include phenol, ethylene glycol, aluminum, and mercury, to name a few. Phenol is a corrosive poisonous compound used as a disinfectant. Skin contact must be avoided, but go ahead and jab some into our baby's arm anyway. Ethylene glycol is used in antifreeze and as a solvent. In vaccines, it is a preservative. But do not worry. Ingestion can only cause central nervous system depression, liver and kidney damage, birth defects and pulmonary edema. Want some more?

Aluminum has been implicated in brain dementia syndromes such as Alzheimer's disease. It is a neurotoxin and poisonous to the respiratory and cardiovascular systems. It can enhance the toxic effects of the mercury in a vaccine as aluminum increases the permeability of the protective blood brain barrier. The blood brain barrier is an extra protective layer of cells that is designed to keep poisons out of our precious brain tissue. Aluminum has the ability to weaken this barrier which enables other toxins to infect the brain.

Mercury is dosed out in the form of thimerosal. Mercury is the third most toxic substance on earth just

---

[16] www.vaccines.plus.com/salk-notstoppolio.html. *The Salk Vaccine and the "Disappearance" of Paralytic Polio.*

behind arsenic and lead. Thimerosal is an organic form of mercury which is far more toxic than the inorganic form associated with fish contamination. Thimerosal is another neurotoxin. It kills brain cells and prevents proper development.

www.youtube.com/watch?v=IHqVDMr9ivo
This link is a video clip from YouTube showing how, in a laboratory, mercury kills nerve cells:

Certain areas of the brain can become damaged from the mercury but the effects will not show up until the infant's development demands use of that specific part of the brain; for example speech or walking. By then the vaccine administration has long been forgotten and doctors are left wondering what happened to this once healthy child. Do we know of a disease that describes a once vibrant, healthy child that all of a sudden, out of nowhere, becomes mentally challenged? One in which this sickness spirals into retardation and a vegetable like state of existence? Ever hear of autism?

This relationship was recently examined on the floor of Congress in which expert after expert came forward and revealed the damaging effects of mercury on our children. An abundance of startling information was exposed during these sessions including the fact that while the EPA sets limits on "safe" levels of mercury, the FDA does not regulate its usage in vaccines.

The EPA's "safe" level of mercury for adults is .1 microgram/kilogram per day. (Please note that is *point* one microgram.) With our child's entry into the world, our baby will receive 30 times that amount in his or her first Hepatitis B shot. By age two, if a child has been submitted to the recommended vaccination schedule, our precious little bundle of joy would have received 237 micrograms of mercury.[17] This is an abomination to our civil liberties and the people who disseminate this kind of medicine should be faced with criminal charges. What kind of perverted mindset must one possess to believe that this mercury poisoning is all in the name of "good medicine"?

Historically speaking, the toxicity of mercury has been known for centuries. The Mad Hatter is not just a character in *Alice in Wonderland*. Mad Hatter Disease was common in England during the 1800s as a mercury based stiffening agent which was used in making the then popular top hats. The vapors from the mercury compound had obvious effects on brain chemistry and function.

The vaccine manufacturers were forced to reevaluate their toxic recipes and, with the help from their personal relations departments, have disseminated the news that mercury would be taken out of the vaccines. However, as late as 2002, five vaccines still contained thimerosal. The 2002 PDR and the package inserts for polio, DPT, influenza, HiB and Hepatitis B disprove any attempt by the vaccine pushers that they have cleaned up their act.

Maybe it just takes a long time for the pharmaceutical companies to cut through all the red tape and change their recipes. The 2004 PDR shows thimerosal was used in the manufacturing of the hepatitis B and the hepatitis A vaccines from GlaxoSmithKline Biologicals. The same can be said for the DPT, polio, hepatitis B combo vaccine from SmithKline Beecham Biologicals. More thimerosal.

Aventis Pasteur Inc. thinks it is a good idea to use mercury in their meningococcal vaccine. Thimerosal lives and stockpiles of vaccines containing this poison exist. You can peruse the FDA's website

---

[17] Tim O'Shea, The Sanctity of Human Blood (San Jose: New West, 2003), pp.111-112.

www.fda.gov/BiologicsBloodVaccines/SafetyAvailability/ VaccineSafety/UCM096228#t3 (table 3, updated June 20, 2012) and find 11 vaccines listed which contain thimerosal. Don't be fooled by blank promises.

> *"There is growing suspicion that immunization against relatively harmless childhood diseases may be responsible for the dramatic increase in autoimmune diseases since mass inoculations were introduced. These are fearful diseases such as cancer, leukemia, rheumatoid arthritis, multiple sclerosis, Lou Gehrig's disease, lupus erthematosus, and the Guillain-Barre syndrome."*
> Robert Mendelsohn

Here's more. The stocks for these vaccines are grown in live protein media. This is done so that the virus for which we will produce the sought after immunity can replicate and then be harvested. A virus needs a protein source to replicate. This protein media includes such scrumptious casseroles as chicken or duck embryo, pig or horse blood, rabbit brain, calf serum, and monkey or dog kidney tissue, to name a few. Once the virus has attached to the protein and replicated, it cannot be separated from the media. The DNA of the virus has intertwined with the protein. No matter how careful the laboratory is in separating the cultured virus from the protein, the protein has become part of the recipe.

This becomes dangerous for two reasons. First, proteins are naturally broken down through digestion into amino acids before being absorbed into the bloodstream. Whole proteins injected directly into the capillary beds of the muscles via the vaccinator's poisonous pen are toxic to the body. The immune system will treat whole protein in the blood the same way that it reacts to other foreign invaders. The whole protein does not belong in the blood and antibodies will be created to try and protect us. Is it possible that our children who are allergic to eggs, chicken feathers, cats, dogs, horses, cows and the like are merely responding to a preprogrammed immune response from these whole protein antibodies? The March 20, 2002 issue of *Dynamic Chiropractic* documented sources that reported vaccinated children are twice as likely to get asthma and other allergy-related symptoms.

Secondly, introducing foreign animal protein into the blood stream exposes any and all diseases of that animal to our own history of viral and bacterial experiences. Whatever suppressed and hidden maladies that there may be in these animals is drawn out when these vaccines are harvested from their protein media. Each of these animals becomes capable of passing on its own version of species specific diseases to us.

Of course the manufacturers will claim that all their vaccine stocks are run through tests and proven to be pure and safe. Do you really think that science has the ability to detect every virus that can or has infected all species of cows, horses, dogs, pigs, monkeys, etc.? The same way that a new nutritional discovery is made every several months (vitamin D is the latest health "discovery") proves that there are elements of life that have existed for eons of time without detection.

The FDA sets limits on how much poison we as humans can "safely" be exposed to without causing permanent damage. As far as I have learned, whether it is the arsenic in our chicken, chlorine in our water, pesticides on our food, or mercury, formaldehyde and aluminum in our vaccines, no poison, no matter how trace, is accepted in the human body to promote health. It is complete lunacy to believe we can inject these deadly toxins into a small child, into anyone for that matter, and in any way improve their health. On paper, the theory of boosting our immune system may sound plausible but in reality only a mad scientist could look at these ingredients and claim that they will promote health.

How prophetic were the words written by Doctor J.M. Peebles in his book *Compulsory Vaccination: A Menace to Personal Liberty,* in 1900, when he penned his thoughts and vision concerning the issue.

"Through this blood poisoning ichor, into which the ruthless lance of the vaccinator is daily dipped, the germs of a legion of diseases assaults the citadel of health, enters the peaceful precinct of home and with the connivance and assistance of the politicians and the legislatures, inflicts upon the little children of the land the barbarous and degrading rite whose curse will spread and multiply through generations yet unborn."

The body has its own innately endowed method of defense and it cannot be enhanced by adding artificial, synthetic pseudo-immunity. If we could create a vaccine from broccoli, carrots, garlic, and Echinacea, I would applaud the effort. The resistance of the body to infection depends on its vitality. If the body is equipped with the proper levels of immune supporting vitamins and minerals, has adequate fresh air, is hydrated with clean water, and is complimented by an animating energy source which is operating without interference, it will resist infection. If our body fails in any of these categories, it will not resist infection. We cannot change the vitality of the body for the better by injecting poison into it. We will only make the body sicker and more susceptible to disease.

Why are booster shots needed if the original vaccine was supposed to create immunity? Is the artificial immunity so fragile and weak that it requires multiple doses to keep it working? If your child has been vaccinated, why should you care if my child goes to school without vaccinations? How can my unvaccinated child spread disease to your vaccinated child if your child is supposed to be protected via immunizations? Are you afraid the immunization in your child won't work?

A pamphlet I obtained from the Iowa Department of Health stated that, "Before vaccines were discovered, childhood diseases took a terrible toll of life and health-the mentally retarded child who was so bright before suffering brain damage from the measles, the baby born blind and deaf because his mother had rubella while she was pregnant, children and adults severely crippled by polio. Even though safe and effective vaccines are available, these tragedies still happen today. In the early 1970's it appeared that childhood diseases were effectively controlled, but the threat of epidemics will grow if children are not protected by immunization."

There are two words in this piece of propaganda that I want to focus in on. They are the words *safe* and *effective*. Edward Jenner's first attempt at producing immunity to smallpox via vaccination was in 1796. During the eight years following Edward Jenner's creation of the smallpox vaccine, the numbers of cases of immunization failures continued to multiply. Jenner advised revaccination and convinced the government and the College of Physicians to support his discoveries. Finally, in 1868, England suffered its worst smallpox epidemic of that century. With 97% of the population vaccinated, nearly 45,000 people died. Where was the protection? After years of opposition to compulsory vaccination laws, England, in 1898, repealed the mandate and no longer forced the issue upon its citizens.

According to the World Health Organization, chances are about fourteen times greater that measles will be contracted by those vaccinated against the disease than by those who are left alone.[18]

A CDC investigation revealed that the source of the December 2000 outbreak of chickenpox in a New Hampshire day care center was a four year old boy who had been vaccinated against chickenpox three years earlier. Not only did a vaccinated boy infect more than half of his day care classmates but 17 of the 25 children who became ill had also been vaccinated. The report is published in the Dec. 12 issue of *The New England Journal of Medicine.* Current studies show the chickenpox vaccine to be only 44% effective so maybe a second dose may be needed. Of course, when the second dose fails to work, the authorities will recommend a third and a fourth dose.

Germany suspended vaccinations for whooping cough in 1975. Gerhard Buchwald, medical doctor, author, and vaccine critic, noted the declining trend in the number of deaths from the disease continued as before.[19] If vaccines were effective we would expect to see just the opposite. In the *New England Journal of Medicine,* July 1994, a study found that over 80% of children under 5 years of age who had contracted whooping cough had been fully vaccinated. A 2012 study led by Dr. David Witt, an infectious disease specialist at the Kaiser Permanente Medical Center concluded that whooping cough occurs more among vaccinated children than children not vaccinated. One could fill an entire book with these kinds of statistics.

> *"Each patient carries his own doctor inside him. We are at our best when we give the doctor who resides within each patient a chance to work."*
> Albert Schweitzer

---

[18] R. Mendelsohn, "The Medical Time Bomb of Immunization Against Disease," *East West Journal,* Nov. 1984, p.49

[19] *The Decline of Tuberculosis Despite "Protective" Vaccination,* p.135. ISBN 3-88721-175-8

Now let's confront the safety issue. Adverse effects from the administration of a vaccine can be obtained simply by reading the package insert or wading through the thousands of pages of a PDR. These can include from the somewhat mild reactions such as rash, fever, night sweats, and swollen extremities to the more severe side effects including vomiting, diarrhea, seizure, muscle spasm, and allergies. Then there is always the possibility of total loss of muscle control, mental retardation, encephalitis, neurological disorders, excessive screaming syndrome, and even death. Do these kinds of warnings come with the purchase of an apple? Will fresh, clean water produce these reactions? What kind of adverse events come with a strong family bond at home?

Adverse events from vaccinations have plagued man since their conception. The 1800s witnessed the smallpox vaccine creating worse epidemics than nature. The 1950s brought us hundreds of victims that succumbed to the paralytic polio by subjection to the Salk vaccine. The 1960s ushered in the measles vaccine that manifested neurological disorders in the very children it was supposed to protect. Let us not forget the swine flu fiasco of 1976 in which the vaccine produced 565 cases of Guillian-Barre paralysis including 30 deaths. The 1980s created a brand new syndrome from the administration of the DPT vaccine; that being the excessive screaming syndrome.

The 1990s heralded in the rotavirus vaccine and its use was suspended after 15 babies had suffered through a life threatening bowel obstruction called intussusception. The 1990s also gave us the Gulf War Syndrome. Nearly 700,000 troops were involved. The Gulf War introduced three new vaccines to its soldiers, none of which were approved due to the immediate necessity of their administration. They were botulism and anthrax vaccines, as well as pyridostygmine bromide which was designed to protect against chemical nerve agents. After reading the twenty three page report filed by a Senate investigation committee, you too will have no doubt left as to the cause of Gulf War Syndrome.[20] There's nothing like a good dose of pyridostygmine bromide, botulism, and anthrax to brighten up the senses.

Heather Whitestone, the 1993 Miss America, was the first ever Miss America crowned with a disability. At 18 months of age, she had a reaction to a DPT shot. The reaction left her deathly ill and consequently left her without hearing. Thank God she didn't come down with diphtheria, pertussis, or tetanus where her body could have fought it off naturally and then develop lifelong immunity. That would have been awful, right? Wrong! I would rather have my child work through the illness of pertussis and come out of it with lifelong immunity to future episodes than to be stricken with deafness for the rest of his or her life. Sorry, I do not see the trade-off.

From www.nutritionreallyworks.com a parent writes, "When my son began his routine vaccination series at age 2 months, I didn't know there were any risks associated with immunizations. But the clinic's literature contained a contradiction: the chances of a serious adverse reaction to the DPT vaccine were one in 1750, while his chances of dying from pertussis each year were one in several million." How have we ever come to accept this trade off?

The DPT vaccine may be the most controversial of all the vaccines. Studies have found a relationship between the vaccine schedules and the incidence of Sudden Infant Death Syndrome (SIDS). Vaccine schedules start at two months and resume at four and six months. Approximately 85% of SIDS cases occur in the period of two to six months with a peak incidence at two and four months. One has to wonder if there is a

---

[20] JD Rockefeller, *Is MilitaryRresearch Hazardous to Veterans' Health?* staff report for US Senate, Dec 8, 1994.

215

correlation between the two. (We also want to have the baby's atlas, the first bone in the neck, checked for misalignment by a competent chiropractor. The atlas can easily become wrenched out of position through the trauma of the birth process. When a baby sleeps on their belly and their head and neck is rotated to one side, the misaligned atlas can create aberrant pressure on the respiratory centers in the brain stem. Breathing irregularities can result.)

One study from the Department of Pediatrics in the UCLA School of Medicine, reported that of the 145 SIDS victims studied, 53 had received their DPT shot in close proximity to their deaths. Twenty seven died within 28 days of their shot, 17 of those within one week, and six within 24 hours.[21]

One can only wonder what the future will bring if we allow vaccination programs to continue to violate Natural Law. No matter how many lives are adversely affected by injecting viruses, foreign proteins, carcinogens, and other poison into our blood, the fires produced are quickly and quietly smothered over by the pharmaceutical-medical blanket never to be heard from again. Vaccines carry no guarantee of safety or efficacy from their manufacturers, distributors, or the government yet they are forced upon us by law. No representing agency will take responsibility for their potential to harm yet they all reap the monetary rewards of their compulsory use. How many people must die or become damaged by vaccines before we say enough is enough? When will science step outside of their ideological box and find a safer way to establish health? When will doctors abide by their Hippocratic Oath and "first do no harm"?

Does all this anti-vaccine information sound like some kind of conspiracy theory? The conspiracy belongs to the AMA, FDA, pharmaceutical companies,

---

[21] Baraff LJ, et al. *Pediatric Infectious Disease,* 1983 Jan-Feb;2 (1): 7-11

and the lobbying groups in government. I have given you nothing but facts concerning vaccines. There is no prejudice or bias embedded in the facts. And I have barely scratched the surface of the vaccine issue. Vaccination is an issue charged with emotion and the decision to vaccinate or not, at least in the court of law, is always based in fear and not reasoning. I fail to see how anyone exposed to this information could possibly accept vaccination as a viable health alternative. Increasing numbers of people, including myself, choose not to believe that we need to infect ourselves with toxic chemicals to keep us healthy. We choose instead to build natural immunity by living wisely and healthfully. We asked to be persuaded by clear evidence and not by force. As far as I can see, the evidence is in nature's favor and not vaccinations'.

"When men differ...both sides ought equally to have the advantage of being heard by the public...for when the truth and error have fair play, the former is always overmatched by the latter."
Benjamin Franklin

An interesting slant on the Hepatitis B vaccine can be found by reading a pamphlet from the Center for Disease Control. The pamphlet leads off with the question, "Why does my baby need Hepatitis B vaccine?" After I read the pamphlet I had to ask myself the same question. The information continued, "You are at risk for HBV if you share needles for injecting drugs, have sex with an infected person, live in a household with someone who has lifelong HBV infection, or have a job that exposes you to human blood." How many of those high risk groups would our newborn baby fit into? Is our baby really at risk here? The greatest incidence occurs in adults from the age of 20-39. The U.S. has among the lowest rates in the world for the disease. According to the 1994 edition of *Harrison's Principles of*

Internal Medicine, hepatitis is not a highly contagious disease. Of those who do catch Hepatitis B, 95% recover completely while acquiring lifelong immunity. So please tell me again why we feel the desperate need to vaccinate all our babies for this?

The medical establishment has done a wonderful job at convincing the public that these childhood diseases are deadly. They are not, in and of themselves, anything more than an innocuous infection. They are no worse than a cold. Pick your illness. The child is sick from one to two weeks depending on several factors. Only the symptoms will vary. The common cold will manifest a sore throat, congestion in the sinuses and chest, and some decrease in energy. This will last for 10-14 days. Measles produces fever, runny nose, and sensitive eyes. A rash soon appears and red spots may cover the entire body. The lymph glands may become swollen. This process will last for 10-14 days. Mumps will bring on swollen parotid glands. Fever, headache, and difficulty swallowing may accompany the mumps. A child with mumps will exhibit these signs of distress for 10-14 days. Are you starting to see a pattern here?

These childhood diseases are benign. I had mumps, measles, and chickenpox as a child. After these illnesses had run their course, I was complemented with natural, life-long immunity just the way nature designed. Childhood diseases are decisive experiences in the physiological maturation of the immune system. These self-limiting diseases strengthen the immune system by creating natural, lifelong antibodies that can recognize any future attack.

Bear in mind that life garners no guarantees as to our life expectancy. Some children will die or be harmed by childhood diseases but not nearly in the numbers used by the drug pushers. These deaths, if examined within a sense of understanding of the Big Picture, are typically more than a case of mumps, chickenpox, measles, or rubella. The trouble comes in the form of additional stress placed upon the still developing immune system. Again, we go back to the basics. Is the baby breast fed mother's milk or bottle fed formula enhanced with synthetic vitamins? Is the baby kept warm or does it sleep in a drafty room? Does the child eat handfuls of refined carbohydrates, like crackers and sugar-filled cereals, or does the child get grapes, blueberries, carrot sticks, apple slices, or raisins for snacks? Is the baby loved and held or is it placed in front of the television and ignored? Has the baby been adjusted by a competent chiropractor? Does the child consume enough Vitamin A, C, D, E, and K in whole food form or does the child get high fructose corn syrup laden ginger ale when he or she is sick? You see, there are many more factors that go into raising a healthy child than merely trying to stimulate an artificial immune response through the administration of poison.

    It is beyond my comprehension to try and understand anyone who has studied the human body on any level and still believes that we need outside synthetic intervention to protect us from infection of innocuous diseases. Take another moment to rethink about the miracle that you are. Remember at conception we are a union of two strands of DNA. From that union springs forth an entire human body. This one cell has multiplied, differentiated, and given us independent life. From one cell we have been equipped with organs completely different in function and form from all others; muscles, nerves, eyes, a liver, neurotransmitters, hormones, intestines, a brain, and so much more. They are all now working in unison to keep us alive. All of these parts are in their proper place making us a perfect whole. And all from one cell! How can a power so magnificent as to create this living, breathing, walking upright, thumb opposing, talking, thinking entity forget to install a system of protection? I am not just referring to any old haphazard, second rate system of protection either. I am referring to an immune system that is just as awe inspiring as the ear is to hearing, the eye is to vision, the lungs is to breathing, and to the heart that never rests.

We do have a defense network installed within us and it is more bewildering than a microscope will ever dissect. Science has tried in vain to tear our immune system apart and they have incorporated fancy sounding names to different cells. They have deduced the cell's supposed functions. However, do not think for one minute that science has even begun to scratch the surface of understanding. Cells in a laboratory are not cells in our body. Our cells are directed by the laws of nature in the grand orchestra we call life. Each one of our cells communicates with all the others via hormones, neurotransmitters, and even through our own thoughts. A laboratory dish will never mimic that. Nature is the master of synthesis, not the scientist. A body in a high state of awareness can adequately comprehend itself and its external environment and thereby adapt to changes imposed upon it. The human body can and will exist in a healthy state if given the proper respect.

I contend that the vaccination program is an initiation to a lifelong addiction to the medicine cabinet. The pharmaceutical establishment is one of the most powerful lobbying groups in the country, grossing billions of dollars in profit annually. With its influence, it has been able to lull the country into a false sense of security. It has been able to convince the government what is best for us and to pass laws supporting their own beliefs. They continue to plot for privilege, place, and power. All done, of course, for the good of the country. The dangers are not found in projected, fear based epidemics. They are found in the vaccines themselves. By artificially immunizing our children, we are poisoning them and denying them the chance of lifelong, natural immunity.

"It is error alone which needs the support of government. Truth can stand by itself."
Thomas Jefferson

Changes in our pattern of living did more to eradicate infectious disease than any vaccine ever did. Smallpox was a disease of small, crowded, filthy cities. The death rate from smallpox was 75% higher in the cities than in the country. The epidemics of eighteenth century Europe were due to the fact that the Europeans had not yet awoken to the necessity of hygiene. With the fall of the Roman Empire, many of the pleasures of life were deigned sinful and unholy. Where once bathing was universal and nakedness was artful, both were shunned. Bodies became not only physically dirty but spiritually dirty as well. Filth was soon universal. Raw sewage was tossed out open windows onto the streets below. Horses left their own special trails of existence on the cobblestone roadways. Narrow streets and poor drainage systems only exacerbated the hapless quality of life. Cesspits abounded and filth accumulated everywhere. It was here where smallpox made its home; in the dead and decaying matter of putrefying compost. Sanitation and lifestyle awareness is the reason smallpox, as well as other contagious diseases, has been eradicated.

Sewage and water treatment plants were developed. Sanitary landfills kept trash, and therefore vermin, away from the populations. Central heating provided escape from drafts and the cold winter air. Iceboxes were used to keep food cool instead of storage in a cellar where it became exposed to varying types of bugs and rats. Straw filled mattresses (Sleep tight. Don't let the bed bugs bite), fly-infested outhouses, and mosquito laden rain barrels were discarded for modern conveniences and, therefore, so too were the modes of transmission for infectious diseases. Germ-carrying rodents and bugs were separated from the masses and these diseases of dirt left with them. As hygiene improved, there was less filth around to allow germs to manifest. (Remember the chapter on The Seed Vs. the Soil.)

By 1900, Dr. Charles Campbell's research (prior research had won him a nomination for a Nobel Prize in containing malaria) determined that the virus associated with human smallpox was spread by bed bugs. Bed bugs infested the straw padded mattresses and were a manifestation of poor sanitation. Their ability to infect was directly related to the victim's level of malnutrition. A malnourished body is not able to mount an effective immune response to infection. Ever hear of him? Probably not. He was another victim of the Medical Inquisition.

Contrast that concept to the inventor of vaccines, Edward Jenner. As part of Jenner's well documented legacy, he observed that the milking maids of dairy farms who had acquired the disease of cowpox from the teats of some cows were not susceptible to the infection of the human smallpox. He concluded that cowpox confers immunity to smallpox. He tried his theory out by inoculating one young boy with cowpox. When the boy did not develop smallpox, the claim was made and history had written another chapter.

A closer look at his legacy exposes a different story. Jenner's conclusions were drawn from one dairy farm. Whether or not milk maids who had contracted cowpox never caught smallpox depended on which farm was studied and who was interviewed. Jenner took one isolated event and created a widespread blanket statement. He also tested his theory on only one person and immediately claimed that the immunity worked. The fact that eight year old James Phipps did not come down with smallpox is irrelevant. He also did not come down with mumps, chickenpox, or syphilis. Does that mean that cowpox also provides immunity to those diseases?

And what about this fact; Cowpox and smallpox

are two entirely different diseases. Cowpox is caused by a virus called orthopox vaccinia and only infects female cows. Smallpox is caused by a virus called orthopox variola and is only found in connection with humans. To imply that cowpox can somehow magically transform itself into smallpox immunity is nothing short of fantasy. Can we grow an orange from the seed of an apple tree? Of course not. How can you grow small pox immunity from a cowpox virus? Now which theory on the origins of smallpox sounds more plausible?

> *"The poetry of the earth is never dead."*
> John Keats

Here are some quick statistics to demonstrate the fallacy and insanity of this "Jenner saved the world from smallpox" illusion. Before 1853, when compulsory immunization was established in England, the highest number of deaths from smallpox in a two year period was about 2000. From 1857-1859 there were over 14,000 deaths attributed to smallpox. From 1863-1865, there were over 20,000 deaths. By 1867, the English Parliament enacted even tougher vaccination laws but found nearly 45,000 people die from smallpox the following year.[22] Where is the protection? Need more? In 1917, after World War I, the United States inoculated some 25 million Filipinos. The smallpox death rate quadrupled shortly thereafter, killing 71,453 of the 162,503 islanders who became infected.

For most people, this information is new and quite unbelievable. History has taught us that Edward Jenner was a great scientist who saved the world from the ravages of smallpox. He is the father of all the other vaccination programs that have supposedly saved millions of lives from other diseases. Why the reason for

---

[22] McBean, E, *The Poisoned Needle*, Health Research, Mokelumne Hills, 1993, p.13.

such contradiction in the biography of Edward Jenner?

The creation of vaccines is a large building block in the foundation of modern medicine. It allowed the medical paradigm to perpetuate through the masses. Jenner's introduction of vaccination was the supposed proof that science could intervene in natural process and manipulate biological outcomes with man-made theories. Man had one-upped nature. Ever since then, science has been trying to outthink Mother Nature by creating a billion dollar industry called pharmaceuticals. Modern medicine will never accept the reality of Jenner's incomprehensible thought process because to do so would invalidate the entire medical profession.

I have read literally dozens of books concerning the vaccination debate. I have researched information in libraries and through the internet. I have studied statistics and learned how to read between the lines of the medical propaganda. It is not my intention here to discuss the vaccination issue ad infinitum. If others wish to further understand the legacy of the mandatory vaccine programs, I recommend www.nvic.org or a quick search on the internet for other websites. Through these sources free thinking citizens can arm themselves with knowledge to confront these drug pushers. One can learn legal steps to take to protect our rights. With a few clicks of the mouse, we can learn how to write a letter of exemption for children to be admitted to school without their shots.

Some states (Arizona, Utah, Arkansas, Idaho, Louisiana, Maine, Texas, Minnesota, Missouri, Nebraska, North Dakota, California, Colorado, Ohio, Oklahoma, Wisconsin, Michigan, Vermont, and Washington) offer philosophical exemptions. Those, of course, are the easiest to obtain. The parents state in writing that they do not want their child vaccinated, and that is that.

The hardest to acquire is a medical exemption. The parents would need to find a doctor who agrees with their choice not to vaccinate. They are out there, but they are few and far between. Your child may also have to have had an adverse reaction to a vaccine to qualify for the medical exemption.

Available to everyone though (except for those living in Mississippi and West Virginia) is the religious exemption. Religious objection may be personal and need not be directed by the tenets of an established religious organization. Parents do not have to be part of a recognized religious organization to claim religious exemption. If school denies religious exemption, they are violating your federally protected civil rights.

This shouldn't be misconstrued as legal advice. I am not a lawyer. I am only offering outlets to investigate the vaccination issue for yourself. All decisions we make pertaining to our freedom of choice are entirely our own responsibility. If we decide to not expose our children to the dangers of mandatory vaccines, we will no doubt be confronted with a litany of opposition. The fight to stand up for our rights will be a long, hard one. School officials, health officials, neighbors, family members, and any group claiming to protect the rights of children will be confronting us with accusations, name-calling, and finger pointing.

We will need to stand by our principles and endure the storm. We may even take it upon ourselves to try and educate these people in the same manner as I have done with this book. Some will listen. Most will not. My final word on this topic is to not let these groups bully us into their paradigm of misinformation. Being strong and committed to our ideals, in the long run, will make us glad we did.

"The question is not whether we die but how we live."
Joan Borysenko

CHAPTER TWENTY

ACUPUNCTURE: NEW AGE MEDICINE IS AGE OLD WISDOM

"The people who oppose your ideas are inevitably those who represent the established order that your ideas will upset."
Anthony D'Angelo

Acupuncture and chiropractic, although appearing rather unique on the outside, are in their effect quite similar on the inside. Albert Einstein's $E=MC^2$ equation stated that matter and energy are one in the same. With chiropractic, the treatment is designed around manipulating matter (our bones) to affect our energy (the nervous system.) Acupuncture, conversely, manipulates our energy (the chi) to affect our matter (the body systems.) Two distinctly different systems now become one workable forum. This relationship between structure and function (another way to describe matter and energy) aides in interfacing chiropractic and acupuncture into complimentary techniques of natural medicine. By rereading the chapter on chiropractic, one can transplant the words acupuncture and chi whenever I have written chiropractic and nervous system. This is not to devalue either modality's place in history or their respective niches in healing. However, anyone with a talent for reading between the lines would note a coarse description of acupuncture overlapping the themes of chiropractic and visa-versa.

This chapter is not written to explain the fundamentals of the application of acupuncture. I am not going to explain the five phases, or the yin yang theory, or the differences in the meridians. If anyone desires to understand the ins and outs of acupuncture, they can obtain that information from an acupuncture clinic in their neighborhood or by reading any number of books on the subject. I will instead try to alleviate some of the stigmas associated with acupuncture and new age medicine as I address some of the disparaging nomenclature associated with it.

One way to degrade the opposition in any forum is to create a negative public relations campaign against them. Simply circulate bogus information or bias, slanted points of view. I do so get a kick out of the old school pundits trying to downgrade the efficacy of acupuncture by referring to it as new age medicine. This label is somehow supposed to invalidate a healing tenet that has sustained a culture through several millennia. This is exactly where acupuncture acquires its own substantiation. How can this style of healing be invalid if it has preserved a continent through eons of time regardless of scientific data? The fact is acupuncture has worked in the past; it works today, and will continue to heal people in the future, with or without FDA or AMA approval. As they say, the proof is in the pudding. Just because one does not understand the makeup of Chinese medicine, does not mean it cannot provide benefits for others.

Acupuncture has been around for at least as long as man has had written language. It has a clearly recorded history of some 2,000 years. Some historians even date acupuncture to be as old as 4,000 years as cave paintings depicting acupuncture type treatments have been discovered. The foundational philosophies that serve as the backdrop for acupuncture are from the Taoist traditions and they are over 8,000 years old. Compare that ancient wisdom, worldly knowledge, profound anecdotal evidence, and irrefutable experience to the mere 200 years of the modern medical approach to health. So just what exactly is so "new" about acupuncture?

If we choose instead to define new age literally as the late 20th century social movement which draws on ancient concepts from the East as well as Native traditions and incorporates them into such themes as holism, respect for Natural Law, spirituality unbound by religious dogma, and metaphysics, then I suppose we could label acupuncture as such. But what is so wrong with that? If that is truly the makeup of new age medicine, why does that make people squirm so? What is it about this new age label that conjures up such opposition? Is it because this alleged new age medicine has not passed the test of scientific research?

Scientific research gave us Acutane to treat acne and low and behold it has been shown to create suicidal tendencies and other psychological instabilities. Scientific research gave us Prozac, Zoloft, Paxil, Wellbutrin, and other antidepressants that now come contained in packaging that warns of suicidal tendencies in children and adolescents. It has been documented that these mind altering drugs can create homicidal ideation as well, though Columbine and the hundreds of other schools ravaged by senseless violence could have just as easily told you that. A quick trip to www.antidepressantsfacts.com will reveal hundreds of cases of school violence linked to our children and pharmaceutical use.

Scientific research gave us the green light on Vioxx which has now been taken off the market due to its high incidence of life threatening side effects. We can thank science for treating asthma with Serevent whose side effects include life threatening spasms in the lungs. How ironic is a drug that creates the very effect it was designed to treat. It was science that directed us to take Crestor for cholesterol only to have many recipients suffer from kidney failure. How quickly have the drugs Clioquinol, Eraldin, Zomax, Osmosin, Flosint, Zelmid, Enkaid, Thalidomide, and Tambocor been swept under the rug to hide them from our memory? Wait. There's more. The safety of Celebrex and other Cox-2 inhibitors (anti-inflammatories that won't irritate the stomach) Has been scrutinized. Even over the counter medication such as Aleve has been implicated in safety issues. Is this where we should all get on our knees and thank science for knowing all there is to know about life. It's looking like folk medicine and new age medicine are not that bad after all.

The history of medical science is littered with failures. I have discussed many of them throughout this book. If scientific proof is the basis for rebuking new age medicine, then that argument has no merit. Let me remind the reader that traditional medicine is the number one cause of death in this country. It is quite clear to me that scientific research does not guarantee any sort of distinction between what is righteous and true and what is not. Scientific relevance is not a marker for the unmitigated proof of reality. Traditional Chinese medicine makes perfect sense within its own paradigm. Obviously, traditional Chinese medicine is not rooted in the same paradigm as America's medicinal system. This does not automatically invalidate it.

Perhaps the uneasy feeling that new age medicine evokes in some people is because this brand of medicine cannot prove innate intelligence, chi, or other energy concepts? Well, can we dissect our heart and find love? Of course not but we know love exists. Can we analyze the seasons and find some internal alarm clock that cues each one to change? Of course not but they change anyway. Prove loyalty, desire, or fidelity. They all exist yet have no measurable quality. Science does not understand these mechanisms but we all have experienced them.

The energies of ultraviolet, infrared, x-rays, and microwaves all existed before science discovered them and created technology to harness them. Now they are an accepted part of our world. What were they before they were discovered? Nonexistent? Can innate intelligence, chi, and love actually have measurable qualities to validate their existence but science hasn't developed technology to measure them yet? Energy exists in many forms. Some energy has been identified and labeled. Some energy still remains a mystery. Why do some cultures accept energy concepts while others do not? Doesn't this point of contention all boil down to the arrogance of the United States standing up to the rest of the world and proclaiming, "We are right and you are wrong"?

Because one body of authority cannot discover answers or cannot understand a concept such as acupuncture does not annul the concept for the rest of the world. Following its own course of diagnosis and treatment, not constraining itself to a class of narrow minded lab coats, acupuncture holds its own as a premier healing art. Unlike the ego of man, acupuncture does not need to be accepted to create a sense of value. It works with or without scientific approval. What would happen to the profitability of modern medicine if it came out tomorrow and declared acupuncture as a viable alternative to drugs?

Let's continue to examine the above definition of new age and try to reason away the rest of your fears. Metaphysics is another one of those words associated with things considered to be new age and therefore it can add to the apprehension of acceptance and understanding. Metaphysics is not the religion of witches and pagans. It is not a word relegated to gypsies and tarot cards. It is not the science of the devil who is trying to undermine "normal" science. These definitions may sound off the wall to some but I have heard them used in regards to chiropractic, acupuncture, and other forms of energy or natural healing.

Metaphysics literally means after the physics. It is the science of being with reference to its abstract conditions as compared to the science of determined values. It is merely everything science can't or has not yet proven. It is a branch of philosophy that examines the nature of reality beyond scientific analysis. Would it make medical minded zealots feel safer if we make it illegal for these philosophers to think beyond the walls of comprehension? Without abstract thinking, we would not have cell phones, satellite television, or computers. No plasma screen TVs, no video games, and no automobiles, no MRI technology, and no airplanes. For these items to exist someone had to think outside the box and dream of a new world. At one point, those technologies had to be considered metaphysical. They were outside the realm of proven science.

Has the power of prayer been scientifically proven? What electronic frequency do prayers travel on? How do prayers work? Does God answer them all or does He have help? No one really knows but there are millions of people who believe in prayer. If prayer has not been scientifically proven, it must be metaphysical.

Angels, ghosts, Ouija Boards, astrology, and Tarot cards have not been scientifically proven so they can be placed in the category of metaphysics. UFO's and Big Foot have not been proven to exist either but there are many people who have experienced that there is indeed "something out there." Metaphysics is simply the "something out there" factor that has yet to be determined. Does it mean these things truly exist as such? No. It means there is "something out there" which cannot be explained. Why does that scare some people? Do they think that science has discovered and explained every phenomenon that will ever be discovered? Doesn't it make more sense to say that one may have a fear of the unknown than it is to say metaphysics is the science of the devil? Would it be more appropriate to say that one may have control issues and because these elements exist outside of scientific analysis one cannot completely control their environment?

The difference between happy tears and sad tears has not been scientifically proven. The state of dreaming is a mystery. Why do we do it? Where does it come from? What do they mean? The genesis of a snowflake distinct from all the other snowflakes ever created cannot be explained. Why do whales beach themselves? Why do some dogs chase cats and others cohabitate peacefully with them? All of these things we know exist but cannot be explained. Why can't there be other elements that exist that cannot be scientifically explained? How about acupuncture and the energy called chi coursing through our body's meridians? Can acupuncture be as real and valid as dreams, snowflakes, and whales? Metaphysics is not witch science for star gazing pagans. Metaphysics is the antithesis of narrow minded tunnel vision. It is the ability to dream of a new and better tomorrow.

"To know that you do not know is the best. To pretend to know when you do not know is a disease."
Lao Tzu

Holism is one of those words that we alternative practitioners love to toss around. Maybe the word holism, within the definition of new age, makes one turn a cold shoulder to reason? Holism is not a satanic word that we must be afraid of. It is not some backwoods offshoot of voodoo. Holism implies interconnectedness with all things. It is a respect for all life in all its forms. It is knowing that every piece of the puzzle is joined explicitly, intricately, and synergistically to each other.

Let's say there is a chocolate chip cookie on the table in front of us. Some may see a tasty snack and nothing more. My holistic perception would see the farmer harvesting the wheat for the flour. I would see the fields the wheat grows in that require sun and rain. I see the fertile soil. I would see the cows that give the milk and the chickens that lay the eggs. I would see the sugar plantation, the bakery and the delivery trucks. I would see interconnectedness ad infinitum. That is holism.

Holism does not separate parts and place them into categories of importance. Holism does not have an hierarchy. The size of an atom is no less or no more than that of a planet. Our finger nail is just as integral as our gall bladder. A spotted owl is as fundamentally a part of the ecosystem as our pet Dalmatian. Celebrities' lives are no more special than yours or mine. Holism respects all that there is and it does not compromise one for another. It is an appreciation of knowing that everything is connected, body, mind, soul, and spirit. Holism is the opposite of arrogance and isolation. It is the acceptance of humility and community. Aren't humility and a sense of community good foundations to raise our children upon? What's so satanic about that?

Respect for Natural Law is an understanding of holism in that the human body, or all of life for that matter, is infinitely more intelligent than the finite thinking of the mind of man. It is the comprehension of the cycling seasons without having to explain them. It is the acknowledgment that food chains are delicately balanced and the extinction of the smallest spider has a profound effect on the stability of the planet. It is a knowing that the human form needs fresh, clean air, pure unadulterated water, and organic whole food nutrition to sustain itself properly. It is knowing that even without man's intervention, life will continue just as purely as it always has.

Natural Law is not an earth worshiping tenet from a leftover, hippie loving cult. In fact, it is the exact opposite. Understanding Natural Law creates an appreciation for the perfection of life as created by a perfect God. Respect for Natural Law denounces food processing, synthetic vitamins, and cocksureness. Comprehension of this concept is having faith and gratitude in divine purpose. Faith and gratitude sound like good tenets to build one's life upon. Natural Law is the function of the planet the way God designed it not the way man thinks it should be. Try as it might, scientific theory will never usurp Natural Law.

"Man did not weave the web of life; he is merely a strand in it. Whatever he does to the web, he does to himself."
Chief Seattle

Is the flinching and twitching some people exhibit with the words "new age" due to the fact that acupuncture does not credit man's ego but rather credits divine wisdom? Is it because this divine wisdom may embrace a non-Christian definition of spirit? Is it because acupuncture does not need a green light from organized religion to understand the sacred creation and maintenance of life?

Spirituality unbound by religious dogma does not mean we cannot practice the traditions of one's faith. It means we understand that there are infinite ways to express gratitude and love for the creation of life. It means the multitude of traditions and rituals are very much a part of one's own religion and are powerful tools for expressing one's appreciation for his or her own being. It means an infinite God cannot be pigeonholed into one finite expression. Every culture on this planet has its own unique styles of clothing, food, and language so why can't they also have a unique way of expressing their spirituality?

The world religions all espouse the existence of one creative force. (Yes, even the Native Americans believed in only one supreme creator.) Regardless of one's religion's uniqueness, within every religion there is a divine message sent to its people via some identifiable messenger. Jesus preached the message of forgiveness. Buddha brought the message of compassion and virtue. Moses carried the Ten Commandments down from Mount Sinai. Love your parents. Don't kill or steal. Don't be envious of your neighbor and don't lie. Confucius spread the virtue of doing what is right not what is of advantage. None of these religions, in their purest forms, teach elitism, hatred, violence, greed, or corruption. Those are ego driven, man-made influences that have built the walls around the world's religions. Once again we see the destructive capacity of man's influence. Can we even imagine a world where these religions practiced what they preached? It would surely look and act completely different from the one we see today.

Unbound spirituality is just that. It is the antagonist of rooted dogma. It is the interaction with the Infinite and the unmitigated belief in the entirety of the Divine. It is believing in and loving all. It is the message sent to us before man's greed for power and domination cleaved us from its unfeigned content. Because our expression of life differs from others does not mean we will rot in hell. It means only that our expression of our life, our spirituality, is mirroring its original, omniscient, omnipotent source.

"This is my simple religion; there is no need for temples, no need for complicated philosophy. Our own heart is our temple, the philosophy is kindness."
Dalai Lama

The belief that new age medicine is somehow evil or unscientific is an unfounded one. It is a statement that someone or some group has programmed us to believe in. We are all in a sense brainwashed into believing or disbelieving certain information. Our entire concept of the world comes from accepting or not accepting other's points of view. Why else would we have Democrats and Republicans? Red Sox fans and Yankee fans? Jay Leno vs. David Letterman? We all live on the same planet yet we all have been raised to appreciate different ideas.

Graduating from a high school in New Hampshire, I learned that the Civil War was brought on because of the actions of the rebel South. I bet kids in the South learn that the Civil War was the fault of the damn Yankees in the North. Who's right and who's wrong? In the Navy, I was taught that the Russian sailors only had one uniform and they rarely washed it. I was old enough and open minded enough then to understand this was the government's way of brainwashing us into believing that the Russians were somehow less human and that they were dirty, second class citizens. I wonder how many of my fellow classmates believed it. I was told in Sunday school that Eve was cast from Adam's rib and therefore men have one less rib than women. This was not a fact taught in any anatomy class I have ever taken since and dissecting cadavers in chiropractic college proved the assumption erroneous as well.

Our minds gather infinite pieces of data throughout our lives. Some we hang on to and make part of our own reality; this is my mother and this is my father. Some we disregard as not true; Santa Claus does not fly around in a sleigh pulled by reindeer. The pieces you have hung on to are different from the pieces I have hung on to. Every person, rich or poor, and every organization, medical or religious, and every culture, industrialized or third world, has its own unique collection of statements, data, and tools to aid in their own definition of the world.

The Christians hang onto the belief that Jesus is the only begotten son of God and he died on the cross for our salvation. Through Jesus is the only way to reach heaven. That is information they have been taught and is part of their fabric of reality. Does that mean the Jews will be condemned to hell? The Jews claim that they are the chosen religion. Does that mean that the Christians will not get into heaven? Who's right? Who's wrong? It seems to me that they both have pretty good marketing plans.

Whether the distaste for new age medicine grows from a scientific or a religious background, neither entity has a proven track record of pre-eminence. Both groups claim dominion over the planet but turn a blind eye to the millions of innocent people they harm and kill. Medicine poisons us with mercury in our fillings and in our vaccines. Wars are waged in the name of God. Medicine creates chemical therapeutics that create dangerous and life threatening side effects. Religion's unyielding dogma fostered The Crusades and the Salem Witch Trials sentencing countless innocent lives to death. Medicine built a country where diabetes, cancer, asthma, allergies, fibromyalgia, and arthritis flourish all the while refusing to accept other healing modalities' points of view. Religion's inability to appreciate an open, thinking mind ushered in The Dark Ages. The purpose of this book is not to debate religion per se or compare corruption between science and religion. It is simply to point out to the reader that no governing body, be it medical science, religion or any other assemblage of authority, holds a patent on reality.

"In religion and politics, people's beliefs and convictions are in almost every case gotten at second hand, and without examination, from authorities who have not themselves examined the questions at issue but have taken them at second hand from other non-examiners whose opinions about them were not worth a brass farthing."
Mark Twain

We, the consumer of life, must take it upon ourselves and weed through all the data placed in front of us. Do not become beholden to any supposed expert. We must discern for ourselves which stimuli are positive and which are negative. We must decide what is true for each one of us. We must make the choices that will ultimately govern our own life. It is not my function to brainwash you or convince you that my ideas concerning health are correct and medicine is wrong. My function is to educate you on the many possibilities you have available to you and help you make the correct decision for yourself. I am merely the shipmate in the crow's nest informing you of approaching hazards and giving you the options to avoid them. Whether we choose traditional medicine or natural medicine, we are ultimately the captain of our ship and must take the information, process it, and steer our ship into a safe harbor.

"...when one side only of a story is heard, and often repeated, the human mind becomes impressed with it, insensibly."
George Washington

CHAPTER TWENTY ONE

LOOK OUT FOR THE BOOGEYMAN

"Neither a man nor a crowd nor a nation can be trusted to act humanely or to think sanely under the influence of a great fear."
Bertrand Russell

There is a phenomenon in this country that is driven by a frenzied media and fueled by profit. It is one that propagates upon our ignorance and our fears making us conform to the standards imposed by others. If we do not act like everyone else we will be labeled as an outcast. This fear of acceptance has denuded our common sense to the degree that we accept the price tag of someone else's perception of life without question. We are led by blind faith, assuming somebody else must know better than we do. Americans have become Pavlovian dogs, programmed to respond in a calculated manner. When we hear about news updates on television, or read them in a newspaper or magazine, we accept it as gospel. Did you hear the latest? Can you believe so and so did that? Isn't the world in such a mess? What are we going to do? Whatever we do, just don't rock the boat.

When the storytellers realize that their audience sits like mesmerized zombies, the stories grow bigger and bolder. And, to add an exclamation to their tales of grandeur, a dose of hysteria gets mixed in. Fear reinforces the implied magnitude of the story. Every year seems to bring heightened surveillance and public warnings of some impending doom. These false impressions of disaster seem to grab the country by the throat and strangle it into a state of unconscious delusion.

Modern history had the country lining up for their shots anticipating the Swine Flu of 1976. The panic over the impending crisis materialized. The flu never did. In 1994, the Hantavirus epidemic was declared imminent. After a few isolated incidences of flu like symptoms, the virus returned to oblivion. The discovery of the Ebola virus of 1995 had the alarm ringing once again and prognosticated the next worldwide epidemic. Where is it now? The summer of 2003 had us in a mania over the West Nile Virus. Every night the news reported the body count of those who had been infected. This new scourge was promoted to the nth degree as the next big killer virus. How much news did you hear about West Nile in the summer of 2004? 2006? Not much at all. West Nile has turned out to be another cursed tale of imminent doom created and propagated by those who would profit from it.

Lest we not forget SARS. Remember the pictures of global panic in which people everywhere were donning surgical face masks? Thousands worldwide were infected, mostly in China. Toronto shut down its borders. If we are going to blame a virus then what about the billions of us who were not infected? Why hasn't there been any news focusing on the rest of us and why we did not succumb to this worldwide health threat? What makes some people immune to these viruses and some people succumb to them is never explored. The priority as dictated by the media is to run and hide from the boogeyman. The vitality of the infected host is never mentioned as a deterrent.

These latest "epidemics" are not due solely to the virulence of a virus gone psycho. There are many other factors well within our control that come into play here. The SARS death rate has been reported at 3-6%, but doubles in polluted cities due to increase in environmental toxins and physiological stress, and rises sharply to 43% for those over the age of 60 (a sector of our population not known for an abundance of exercise or healthy food choices.)

In 2012, West Nile Virus has been resurrected. Science wants us to believe a mosquito bites an infected bird and then bites a human thus transferring the virus. Remember our eagle soaring high in the sky looking down on both sides of the mountain. Researchers Jim West and David Crowe have been vigilant in trying to expose what they believe is the WNV fraud. Mr. West has also researched the cause of polio and found it not to be a virus at all. His conclusion is that polio was caused by industrial pollution, most conspicuously by DDT poisoning. DDT poisoning mainly came from cows eating foods that had been contaminated with the DDT. This then showed up in high concentrations in the milk and ice cream products. Like the cause of polio, Mr. West believes WNV is not a virus but a cellular response to environmental poisoning.

Birds (as well as other animals) are feeling the effects of man's continued assault on this planet with toxic chemicals. When a bird dies and it is found to have antibodies to a virus, it does not mean that virus killed it. If I have a heart attack and upon autopsy it is revealed that I had antibodies to chickenpox, it does not mean I died from chickenpox. I had a heart attack. We all carry many viruses inside us and we do not die because of them. There are other causes of bird deaths.

West asserts that much of the sickness associated with WNV is caused by exposure to record high levels of summer air pollution, exacerbated by the gasoline additive MTBE (methyl tertiary butyl ether). The recent epidemic of bird deaths and the WNV "epidemic" could be a warning regarding refinery pollution. Industrial air pollution and its role in WNV are never addressed on a large media-wide scale though virtually all such epidemics have occurred downwind from oil refineries. We continue to overlook what may be too obvious a solution due to our acceptance of the dominant virus theory. Can West Nile Virus not be the cause of disease but rather the result of a polluted ecosystem? Naw! That's too easy.

"No great epidemic has ever evolved divorced from major socio-political upheaval."
Leonard Horowitz

The vast majority of people affected by these pathogens are old, immunologically weak, or infirmed. They are the same people that would have been susceptible to the multitude of other viruses or bacteria present in our environment. They are people whose immune systems are depleted to begin with for any number of reasons. They are, shall we say, ripe for the picking. No matter which innocuous little germ that sweeps through, these people would most likely fall victim anyway: A classic example of survival of the fittest. It is not the strength of the virus that is to be feared. It is the strength of our immune system that needs to be promoted. So how fit are you?

The world is awash in the belief that HIV causes AIDS. After reading Peter Duesberg's book, *Inventing the Aids Virus*, as well as several other books on the subject, I have some questions concerning that proclamation. Why has the latency period of HIV been expanded from 10 months to 10+ years? Is it to keep the infected numbers high and propagate an epidemic? Latent viruses defy the laws of virology. Viruses can't hang around and wait to cause damage ten years later. Viral infection creates antibody production and antibody activity is immediate in its response. No virus can loiter around undetected. We all know this because the hallmark used by medicine for HIV infection is not an active virus but rather antibodies to the virus. Why do antibodies neutralize every other virus except HIV? HIV's genetic makeup is no "smarter" than a cold virus. Its genetic makeup is no more specialized than any other retrovirus. There is no secret gene hiding on a remote chromosome underneath an undetected strand of amino acid. Are we to believe then that this innocuous virus is somehow tricking our immune system when no other more powerful virus could?

We are told HIV infects T cells within the immune system's arsenal and eventually destroys them. A low T cell count is another hallmark of HIV infection. If HIV kills the cells it has infected, how can it continue to live and spread? No other virus kills its host. If the host cell dies, so does the virus. The viruses want the cells to not only live but to keep on regenerating. Without a cell to leech onto, the virus dies - no cell, no home. Also to note, T cells replicate 500 times faster than HIV can infect. How, then, does HIV ever get the upper hand? It can't and that is why humans can show HIV antibodies. Our immune system has worked perfectly. If HIV is an immunosuppressant, how can it be blamed for non-immunosuppressant diseases relegated to the AIDS definition such as dementia and wasting syndrome? Isn't AIDS just another name for a grouping of some 25 diseases that have already existed?

Several factors came together at the same time to promote this propaganda. The virus hunters had spent ten years searching for a virus that causes cancer and failed. Simple logic could have been used here and saved lots of time and tax money. Viruses are contagious. Cancers are not. With this failure looming over their heads, the virus hunters really needed a rally. In 1980, technology for counting T cells emerged and needed a disease to practice on. Once a few homosexual men showed up with strange sets of symptoms, their T cells were counted and the game was on. At first AIDS was labeled a gay issue. Then it grew into an illicit sexual contact issue. Then HIV showed up in some blood banks and hemophiliacs were suddenly at high risk. The initial mode of transmission was reported to be from the gay community, spread through anal sex and then contaminated blood donations.

Though political correctness now has the country awash in gay awareness, AIDS is still likened to the gay community albeit under everyone's breath as to not offend. If we are to believe in this assumption, where are the epidemics within the group of heterosexuals that partake in anal sex? I do not mean to be graphic here, but anal sex is anal sex no matter who's giving and who's receiving. Are we to believe that HIV is smart enough to distinguish between homosexual and heterosexual anal sex acts? No other virus is so discriminatory.

"More than 500 of the world's most prominent scientists are questioning the AIDS hypothesis. Their number is growing daily."
Robert Willner

There are too many variables in the HIV theory that do not make sense. No one bothered to explore other options in this condition of immunosuppression. (Or, rather, other options were not allowed into the public arena.) What other ideas are out there? Let's take a look at the "high risk groups" and see if there isn't another explanation for AIDS. We have already mentioned the gay community. Also included in the high risk group are prostitutes, drug users, hemophiliacs, and several African third world countries. Pretend for just one moment that HIV never existed. How can these vastly different groups become connected through immunosuppression? (Keep in mind; no one is debating the condition of AIDS, more appropriately called immunosuppression. The debate is whether or not HIV can cause it.)

Starting with the gay community, we find a subculture that sniffs amyl nitrates. For whatever psychological delinquencies these drugs may hide, these poppers help to relax muscles, especially the anal sphincter, allowing for easier penetration. This group of nitrates is a toxic immunosuppressive agent. A habitual dose of these can cause the immune system to be virtually destroyed, leaving someone with a low T cell count and no protection from other opportunistic pathogens. The February 12, 2005, CNN Headline news offered a piece concerning the rise of AIDS within the gay and bisexual community. They continued with (here's the interesting part that went over everyone's head) "especially those who use crystal-meth." The link here with gay men and AIDS is not HIV but rather immunosuppression via illicit drug use. Having antibodies to HIV does not mean that one has AIDS. It means you have been exposed to a virus and your body has created antibodies to it. You are now as protected as every other person exposed to every other virus.

So what happened to the gay man with HIV who does not partake in the practice of sniffing poppers? Every virus that has ever latched onto us has left its trail of existence within us. HIV is no exception. Many people have been exposed to HIV as they have been exposed to other viruses throughout their life. Antibodies to HIV do not equate to AIDS. What does happen, though, is the mind is filled with the idea and is converted from an "I enjoy life" mindset to "I'm going to die" mindset. The mind is a powerful tool in healing. The placebo effect proves that. The medical establishment then wants to put the infected person on AZT. AZT was initially developed as a drug to help fight cancer but was found to be too toxic for the body. After being shelved for many years, it found a resurgence of sorts in combating an illness that had no medicine. AZT is highly immunosuppressive. Once a deadly mind set and toxic AZT combine to wipe out the immune system, the self-fulfilled prophecy of HIV causing AIDS is manifested and the gay man passes on.

How about prostitutes and drug users? Do they transmit HIV through contaminated needles and illicit sexual activity? (Remember, even if they did, HIV antibodies neutralize the virus 500 times faster than HIV can infect). Aren't these two groups of people subject to self-imposed immunosuppression through their own lifestyles? Drug users and prostitutes are not known for their healthy habits. Their daily routines are filled with poor food choices, if they eat at all, no exercise, no family bonding, no concern for hydrating their bodies with fresh water, and may very well live in squalor. This is a stereotype I know but it is also the reason why not all drug users and prostitutes fall to immunosuppression. Immunosuppression is immunosuppression and it does not require the existence of a wimpy, fragile virus.

> *"The only thing we have to fear is fear itself."*
> Franklin Delano Roosevelt

How did hemophiliacs get on the high risk group list? Anyone receiving a whole protein source from another human being needs to take immunosuppresive drugs for life. This includes organ transplants as well as blood transfusions. To keep our body from rejecting the foreign tissue, to keep our antibodies from mounting an attack on this foreign protein, the recipient will, for the rest of his or her life, become immunosuppressed from drug therapy regardless of HIV infection. Here we can clearly see the linear equation of reductionism working once again. Hemophiliac + immunosuppression + HIV antibodies = AIDS. I believe the alternative explanation above is more valid and is in line with the "Big Picture".

This leaves us with the last group-the African third world countries. In the 1970s, famine was to blame for the wasting syndromes we saw on television. Today, the very same situation, the very same wasting syndromes, is blamed on HIV. Nothing has changed. The exception is that today if a starving, wasting African has HIV (antibodies), then the world hears about the crisis and sees him dying of AIDS. If the African does not have HIV (antibodies), then nobody is notified and he dies quietly from starvation. Starvation is starvation, whether in 1970, 1980, or today. HIV has no bearing on starving Africans. We would do the world a favor if we found a way to feed these people instead of wallowing in our inability to create a vaccine and save the world from an invisible threat.

Do these explanations of immunosuppression sound more plausible than a super-virus, never before seen, that can distinguish between heterosexual and homosexual anal intercourse, can trick the immune system into producing antibodies that do not work, that can proliferate even though it kills the very host that it must use to live in, and can cause some diseases that have nothing to do with immunosuppression even though immunosuppression is its forte? AIDS is immunosuppression brought on by illicit drug use, starvation, or immunosuppressive pharmaceuticals and has nothing to do with an innocuous viral infection. Finding people with HIV and AIDS congruently is coincidence rather than causation. The cause of AIDS is immunosuppression regardless of HIV infection.

Legionnaires' disease is another example of misplaced blame for illness. After attending a bicentennial convention in the Bellevue Stratford Hotel in Philadelphia, hundreds of conventioneers came down with severe and sometimes lethal pneumonia. In its wake, Legionnaires' disease left 221 ill and 34 dead. The Center for Disease Control eventual proclaimed the newly found bacterium Legionella Pneumophila. This bacterium found in the air conditioning ducts was labeled the culprit and the country accepted the findings without question.

Remember Koch's postulates pertaining to the germ theory. The germ must be present in every case of the disease. In this case, 10% of the conventioneers affected were never infected by the bacterium. To add more doubt to the equation, the bacterium is so ubiquitous that between 20-30% of the population has already been exposed and infected without any demonstrable signs or symptoms. If Legionella Pneumophila found in the air conditioning ducts is to be named as the culprit here, why didn't everyone staying at the hotel come down with symptoms? Are the bacteria selective in its attack or were there people in the hotel that had immune systems strong enough to protect them?

Bypassing the linear equation of reductionism and thinking in holistic terms, one would ask the following questions: Could these conventioneers have been victims of their own abuse? How old were they? How much partying did they do while in attendance? Can the cigarettes, smoking, and alcohol drinking associated with conventions and seminars deflate the immune system's ability to defend? Did these conventioneers have prior health risks such as heart, lung, or kidney disease? Were these people already susceptible to opportunistic infection? The answer to all of these questions is yes.

This is not to say that we should haphazardly run through the streets naked without a care in the world. These health threat warnings should not be ignored but I do believe we need to apply a sense of decorum before we proclaim the end of the world is near. We need not cower under these frantic public warnings and heightened surveillance. There needs to be a balance between fear-based propaganda and complete disassociation from reality. I, for one, will not cower from the alarmist rhetoric. I will not let fear tactics rule my decisions. I will instead choose to keep my body in a state of awareness ready to adapt to changes in the environment.

> *"Man is part of nature, and his war against nature is inevitably a war against himself."*
> Rachel Carson

Pain is the result of disharmony. It is brought forth from a body that cannot comprehend the changes in its environment and adapt appropriately. Health is just the opposite. Comfort is achieved when the body understands its place within the Big Picture and can adapt itself with ease to any and all changes posed upon it. Natural medicine works with our body's inherent healing mechanisms. Our bodies can be reset and renewed when deficits are confronted. I choose better quality foods, drink clean water, exercise, and chiropractic adjustments. That is the best medicine anyone can prescribe.

Life is analogous to a giant jigsaw puzzle. Seen from the untrained eye suffering from tunnel vision, the puzzle can appear to be intimidating and complex. The many pieces lay out before us in a mass of dissimilar shapes and unconnected colors. How could anyone align these pieces of life to reveal the pattern inherent in the jigsaw puzzle? If we wait long enough, a neighbor or relative will come to visit and see the puzzle spread out on our table. They too will stare at the pieces in amazement. Maybe they will even join a few pieces together making the picture of health a bit more clear. This is the friend who tells you that glucosamine sulfate is good for your arthritis. It is a tiny piece of the puzzle but still does not complete the entire picture.

There are, however, those of us who are not tyrannized by the mysteries of the jigsaw puzzle. We see how the pieces all fit together. We see the patterns inherent in the design. With just a little bit of time and some creative license we can master the analogy and reveal the ease at which the pieces all fit together, perfectly and effortlessly. The picture on the puzzle, the picture of life, exposes itself without prejudice. It imparts its secrets without remorse. It is more than happy to let us in and play the game. We begin to see that there is a place for medical necessity, as there is a place for everything, but there is a larger part of the puzzle reserved for common sense and its application. The puzzle of life is only difficult if we study one piece at a time separate from the original whole picture. Step back and observe the entirety of the offering and the colors and shapes of the puzzle pieces will tell us exactly where they need to be placed.

I claimed previously in this book that there are no experts and that includes me. Your best course of action right now is to not accept anything I have written. Investigate my statements for yourself. Prove me right or wrong but, more importantly, prove to yourself that there is more than one way to interpret this world and no body of intelligence holds a monopoly on reality.

The natural processes involved in sustaining life need to be nurtured and supported. The more man tries to rewrite God's instruction manual the more frustration and confusion he will encounter. Resisting the will of the Infinite is fruitless. Working within the realm of infinite possibilities is fruitful. We cannot win a fight against the divine wisdom of life any more than we can stop the sun from rising in the East or stop the birds from chirping.

The bottom line in medicine should be focused on whether or not the patient gets well, not on who will financially benefit from a specific course of treatment. Medicine cannot single handedly rule out options only because these options offer success from which medicine cannot profit. The foundation of any healing modality should be dedicated to improving the quality of life of the very people it represents. Well-meaning doctors are often unintentionally causing harm to people by ascribing to the outdated paradigm of Western medicine and the germ theory. Medicine cannot succeed if its focus is zeroed in on elitism, power, greed, or supremacy. Healing is not about ego driven prestige or an authoritative stance bullying clients into submission. Healing is a public service. It is a calling from the heart not the wallet. Healing must first come from a compassionate mind and all else will secondarily follow.

"All you need is love"
John Lennon and Paul McCartney

Made in the USA
Charleston, SC
07 April 2016